ALTERNATIVE ANSWERS TO

ARTHRITIS
& RHEUMATISM

Contents

Introduction

Many people regard arthritis as a disease of elderly people, but this is far from the truth. Arthritis can strike at any age, in the thirties, twenties – even in childhood. This is all the more reason to adopt a positive attitude to seeking out effective treatments for the illness. The 20th century has seen considerable advances in the treatment of arthritis. There is no need for anyone now to contemplate a diagnosis of arthritis with foreboding, or the fear that will mean spending the rest of their life in a wheelchair.

This book examines the many different choices for treatment and for the relief of pain that are open to people who suffer with arthritis. It considers what orthodox medicine has to offer – namely medication, physiotherapy and surgery. It look at all those complementary therapies that are readily available and selects those that are the most appropriate for arthritis sufferers. In addition, it analyses how we live our lives from day to day, with a view to making every aspect of everyday activities easier for arthritis sufferers to cope with.

The last 10 years have seen enormous leaps forward in the treatment of arthritis. It is, therefore, interesting to consider how treatment might be approached in the future. There are many areas, for example, where we know that treatments will change and develop.

• Some conventional and well-known surgical techniques are now outmoded – the trend in surgery, for example, is no longer to repair a joint, but to replace it.

• Joint replacement surgery is currently facing two great challenges. The first is a need to develop longer-lasting joints; the second is to find more

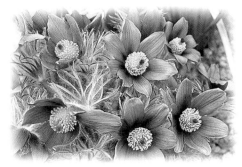

effective ways to attach artificial joints to the bones. Only when both of these challenges have been met will the need for a second joint replacement in a lifetime be eliminated.

• Medication will be become more and more specific so that side-effects are fewer in number and less severe in nature. The pharmacological industry has described such medication as "magic bullets".

• Complementary therapies will probably become even more popular. Some of them are already offered by family doctors and hospital pain clinics, and some are covered by health insurance schemes.

Many people are already familiar with the benefits of massage, osteopathy, acupuncture, herbalism and homeopathy, but what of the newer complementary therapies? For people with arthritis, gentle therapies such as t'ai chi and colour therapy can be recommended without reservation. If you have not tried one or more of the complementary therapies already, it is worth reading chapter 2 right away.

Many people with arthritis complain most bitterly of the pain associated with the illness. Most people can gradually learn to cope with disability, or even immobility, but pain is a constant source of stress, fatigue, depression and frustration. For this reason, most of the therapies, treatments, environmental and lifestyle modifications recommended in this book are those which contribute the most to the control and relief of pain in arthritis.

The future for arthritis sufferers is full of hope – this book will help you to make the most of what is available to control and treat your arthritis.

How to use this book

This book works in several ways. If you read straight through you will understand what arthritis is, how complementary and conventional treatments may help arthritis sufferers, and what you can do on a day-to-day basis to manage both the condition and the pain associated with it. Alternatively, follow the "Find out more" references throughout the book to learn all you need to know about a specific aspect of your condition.

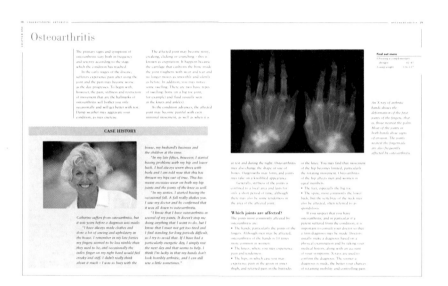

1 Chapter One discusses the different conditions that fall under the "arthritis" umbrella, explains how common arthritis is becoming and the groups most affected, and looks at the current state of knowledge on the causes of arthritis.

2 Chapter Two looks at those complementary therapies that might be of help to arthritis sufferers. These include gentle movement therapies such as t'ai chi which enable you to maintain and improve mobility, as well as therapies to help relieve pain, such as acupuncture or herbal medicine. In each case the philosophy behind the therapy is detailed and its relevance to arthritis sufferers explained.

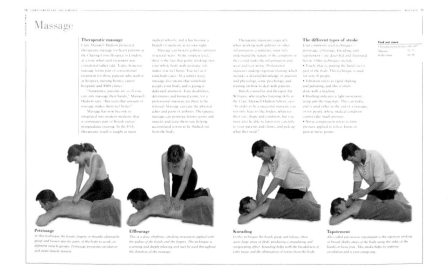

3 Chapter Three considers the conventional approach to arthritis treatment and care. These range from practical therapies, such as physiotherapy or occupational therapy, targeted to your individual requirements, to surgery. Joint replacement, for example, offers increased mobility, freedom from pain, and an enhanced quality of life.

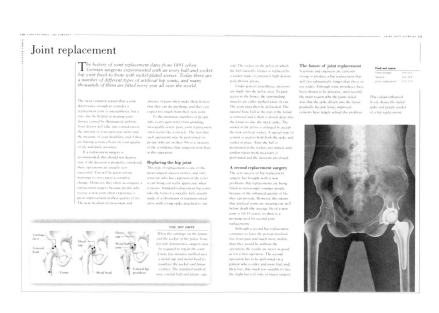

4 Chapter Four deals with the practicalities of living with arthritis. This covers not only such subjects as how to perform everyday tasks, but also considers how diet and exercise can contribute to your quality of life, and how the pain of arthritis can be brought under control, day and night.

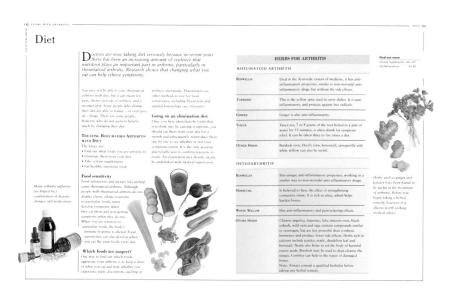

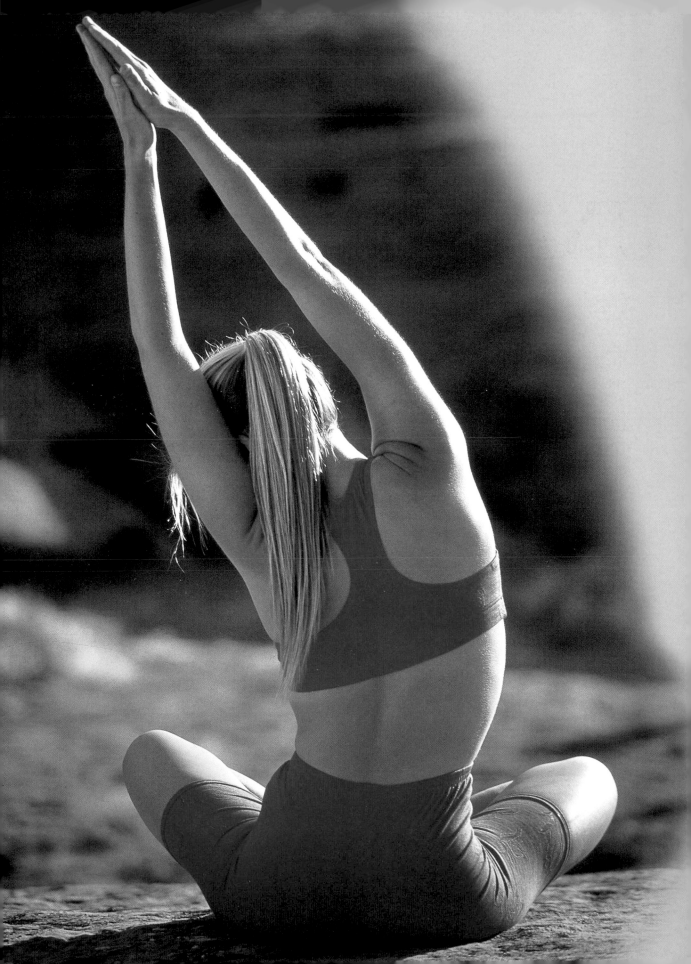

1
UNDERSTANDING

ARTHRITIS

The skeleton is a jointed framework that supports the body and enables it to perform a fantastic range of movements – these are in turn controlled by muscles, tendons and ligaments attached to the bones. A joint is the point where bones meet and move against each other. The human body comprises more than 200 joints, and the principal ones are in the elbows, hands, hips, knees, feet and spine.

Arthritis may develop in any one, or more, of the joints. This common condition is defined as pain, stiffness or swelling in or around a joint that persists for more than two weeks. Given that there are over 200 types of arthritis, it is easy to see why arthritis plagues so many people.

What is arthritis?

*T*he word arthritis literally means "inflamed joint". However, the term does not exclusively refer to the inflammation of a joint. Arthritis may also indicate a joint that is injured, strained, infected, damaged or worn.

When any joint in your body is affected by arthritis, you experience considerable discomfort and pain as a result of the nerves in the joint sending pain messages to the brain. The smooth functioning of the joint starts to break down in an unhealthy or ageing joint.

In osteoarthritis, the cartilage – the fibrous tissue covering the ends of bones – becomes thin and flaky and begins to split. The bone underneath thickens and starts to project at the edges of the joint, reducing the degree of movement. Fluid in the joint increases, leading to swelling, stiffness and pain. The capsule encaseing the joint is stretched. In severe osteoarthritis the cartilage may wear away completely, exposing the bone. Chalky deposits of crystals may form in the bone and can break off and float around in the fluid. The joint may become permanently deformed.

In rheumatoid arthritis, inflammation starts in the membrane surrounding the joint (the synovium), which then thickens and begins to occupy the space within the joint. The inflammation spreads to the rest of the joint capsule, and the ligaments and tendons that surround and support it become stretched, so the joint itself may become unstable. If the inflammation remains unchecked, the cartilage in the joint will shrink and the exposed ends of the bone become eaten away, leading to deformity.

The joints of the body vary widely in their structure. Some, like the hip and shoulder, allow movement in all directions. Others, such as the elbow, move only backward and forward. In the spine the vertebrae have even less independent movement, and they are jointed without a capsule or any lubricating fluid. This leaves the disc of cushioning cartilage between them with an even more crucial role to play; this is why back pain is the most widespread and intractable form of joint pain that troubles human beings.

Types of arthritis

Arthritis takes a number of forms. The most common types are osteoarthritis, rheumatoid arthritis, and gout; these are described in more detail from page 16. Some less common forms of arthritis are described on pages 26–29.

Types of arthritis can be grouped according to the following general causes.

Wear and tear

Degenerative types of arthritis includes osteoarthritis, the most common form. Joints, just like the moving parts of any machine, wear out and perform less reliably with heavy use and with the passage of time. The joints of the human body simply wear out. You may get arthritis as you become older because your cartilage is the type that becomes thin and flaky with age, or because you have exposed your joints to heavy use, perhaps on the sports field, or you may have imposed undue strain on them by loading them with too much body weight. Another possibility is that one of your hip joints is subjected to excessive wear through one of your legs being longer than the other. This is not uncommon.

Inflammation

In inflammatory types of arthritis, of which the most common is rheumatoid arthritis, the cause of the inflammation is often unknown. It is possible that the inflammation is sparked off by a virus. This may trigger the body's own defence mechanisms to turn upon themselves and perpetuate the inflammation even in the absence of any harmful agent. Ankylosing spondylitis is an example of inflammatory arthritis.

Breakdown in body chemistry

The most common of these diseases is gout, in which a joint becomes inflamed because the body fails to flush away harmful crystals of uric acid that form inside the joint, causing intense pain.

Other types

Some types of arthritis are a combination of both inflammation and wear and tear. Arthritis can also be caused by bacterial or viral infection.

WHAT IS RHEUMATISM?

The word rheumatism describes any of the several disorders – including fibrositis and polymyalgic rheumatica – characterized by inflammation of connective tissues, such as muscles, joints and tendons. Common symptoms include pain and stiffness. Some conditions such as rheumatoid arthritis are a combination of rheumatism and arthritis.

JOINTS AFFECTED BY ARTHRITIS

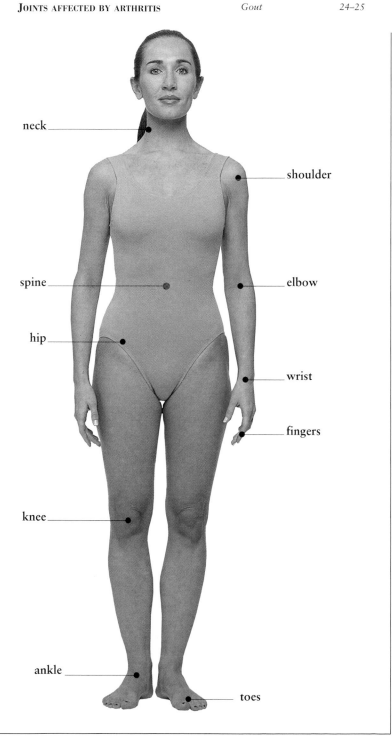

neck — shoulder — spine — elbow — hip — wrist — fingers — knee — ankle — toes

How common is arthritis?

*O*f *the world's population, 90 per cent will eventually develop some form of arthritis. In a number of cases, however, arthritis may cause little trouble because with increasing age most people make fewer demands on their bodies.*

Arthritis is often thought of as a sign of ageing, although it can affect young as well as old people. In fact, arthritis is one of the most common diseases in humans. To give an idea of how prevalent arthritis is, take this figure as just one example: in the United States, 285,000 children suffer from arthritis pain every day.

Records in the United Kingdom show that around 20 million people suffer with arthritis, 8 million of whom consult their doctor for treatment. Osteoarthritis is responsible for 5 million of those 20 million sufferers, with rheumatoid arthritis affecting a further 1 million

individuals. Some 15,000 children are affected by juvenile arthritis.

In the United States, which has one of the most diverse ethnic populations, nearly 40 million Americans (one in seven) have some type of arthritis. (This is projected to rise to almost 60 million by 2020.) Of these, approximately 23 million women of all ages are affected by arthritis. Juvenile rheumatoid arthritis affects 61,000 girls, representing 86 per cent of all cases. In other countries, where similar statistics are available, the proportions of instances have proven to be similar.

The chart below categorizes the number of arthritis sufferers in the United States by the types of arthritis they have. It includes only the most common types of arthritis, accounting for over 23 million people. However, other, less common, forms of arthritis account for more than 16 million people.

* Fibromyalgia, strictly speaking, is a form of rheumatism, rather than arthritis.

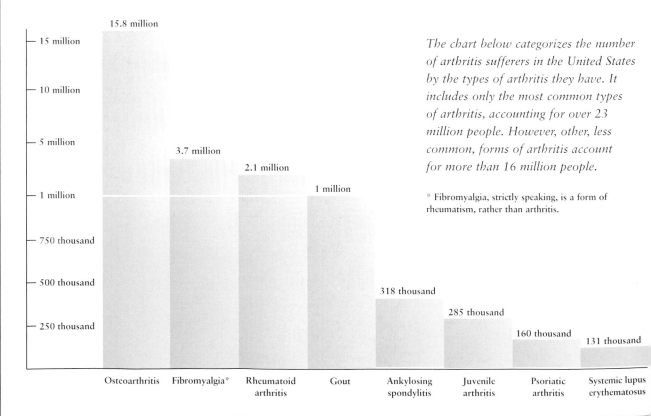

Osteoarthritis	15.8 million
Fibromyalgia*	3.7 million
Rheumatoid arthritis	2.1 million
Gout	1 million
Ankylosing spondylitis	318 thousand
Juvenile arthritis	285 thousand
Psoriatic arthritis	160 thousand
Systemic lupus erythematosus	131 thousand

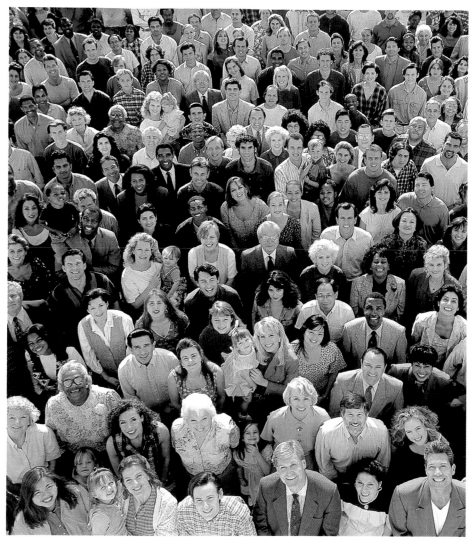

Find out more

What is arthritis	12–13
Causes of arthritis	30–37
Living with arthritis	134–153

Arthritis affects people from all walks of life – no matter what their age, gender, ethnicity or social background. Worldwide, as many as nine out of ten people are affected by some form of the disease.

What are the implications?

The financial implications to health services and health insurance companies are serious. There are also costs for employers who lose money due to absenteeism, either from lost production or by hiring replacements. Every year, arthritis costs the American economy some $54.6 billion in medical care and indirect costs such as absenteeism. It also, obviously, affects the ability of parents or grandparents to enjoy fully children's early years.

Arthritis is the most common cause of disability in the Western world. The disease limits everyday activities – such as getting in and out of bed, dressing, climbing stairs and even walking. Arthritis may lead to reduced mobility, loss of employment, breakdown of social and marital relationships, chronic pain, fatigue and depression. Severely disabled sufferers from arthritis may need support from visiting carers, who can clean or help with shopping, or they may need full-time nursing care.

Osteoarthritis

*O*steoarthritis is the most common form of arthritis, and affects mainly people of middle age and older. The sites usually involved are the neck, lower back, knees, hips and joints of the fingers. The big toe may be affected by osteoarthritis, but this should not be confused with gout.

Nearly 70 per cent of people over the age of 70 have evidence of osteoarthritis that can be seen on an X-ray. However, only half of these people develop symptoms of the disease. In addition to developing in ageing joints, osteoarthritis may occur in joints that have been previously injured or subjected to prolonged heavy use, and in joints that have been damaged by prior infection or inflammatory arthritis. People who suffer from osteoarthritis experience pain and loss of function of the affected joints.

What causes osteoarthritis?

Osteoarthritis results from the gradual degeneration of the cartilage that surrounds and cushions the affected joint.

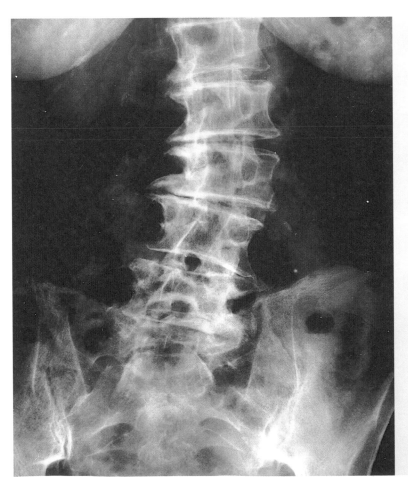

DISCS AND VERTEBRAE

The spine is made up of blocklike bones called vertebrae that sit one on top of the other, cushioned by cartilage in between the bones. Normally the spine runs straight down the centre of the back. The spine (left) of an elderly woman has a prominent lateral curve, or scoliosis, in addition to signs of advanced osteoarthritis. Scoliosis may occur through one leg being shorter than the other, or when pain in the back or legs causes a person to overcompensate by leaning to one side. In addition to a thinning of the cartilage between the bones, osteoarthritis is characterized by the formation of bony projections, or osteophytes, which may appear almost to form a bridge between adjacent vertebrae. (These are visible to the left of the five lowest vertebrae in this X-ray.)

Healthy cartilage that covers the end of the bone in a joint is normally very smooth, strong and flexible. In osteoarthritis, however, this gradually becomes pitted, rough and brittle. There are many causes of cartilage loss.

The thin layer of cartilage at the end of the bones acts as a shock absorber and helps the joint to move. The joint is surrounded by a membrane called the synovium, which is rich in blood vessels and nerve endings. In healthy joints the synovium nourishes and protects the joint and produces fluid – known as synovial fluid – which lubricates the joint.

As the cartilage wears away, the bone beneath thickens and grows outward, thus enlarging the joint. It can also form spurs at the edges of the joint – these are known as osteophytes. These spurs are partly responsible for the knobbly appearance of hands that you sometimes see in older people who are suffering from osteoarthritis.

Osteoarthritis may take many years to develop, and it usually forms in one joint – most often a load-bearing joint – at a time. In some people it produces little more than some stiffness, while in others the disease can cause considerable discomfort and disability.

Is it hereditary?

Some kinds of osteoarthritis are known to be hereditary, including the common form causing enlargement of the first finger joint – these outgrowths are known as Heberden's nodes, after the British doctor who first identified them. Here a specific genetic abnormality, which may be passed from mother to daughter, in particular, has been found. This abnormality causes a change in one of the amino acids (the basic building blocks

of all proteins), which causes cartilage to deteriorate prematurely. Current research focuses on this genetic abnormality as well as new methods of studying cells, chemistry and the function of cartilage.

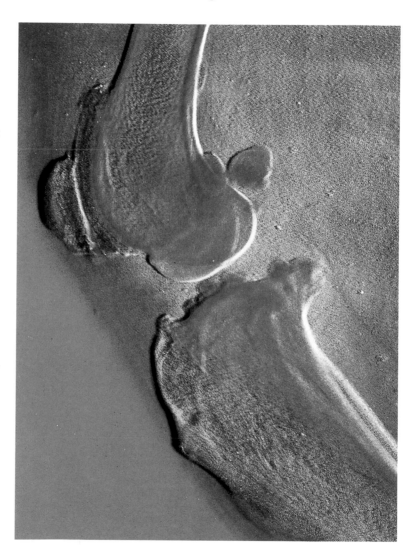

In this severe case of arthritis of the knee, an X-ray shows that the cartilage lining of the thigh bone, or femur (top), and the tibia (bottom) has been eroded. It is also possible for the bone itself to start to erode; here, a fragment of bone (left of the femur) appears to have broken away.

Osteoarthritis

The primary signs and symptoms of osteoarthritis vary both in frequency and severity according to the stage which the condition has reached.

In the early stages of the disease, sufferers experience pain after using the joint and the pain may become worse as the day progresses. To begin with, however, the pain, stiffness and restriction of movement that are the hallmarks of osteoarthritis will bother you only occasionally and will get better with rest. Damp weather may aggravate your condition, as may exercise.

The affected joint may become noisy, creaking, clicking or crunching – this is known as crepitation. It happens because the cartilage that cushions the bone inside the joint roughens with wear and tear and no longer moves as smoothly and silently as before. In addition, you may notice some swelling. There are two basic types of swelling: bony (in a big toe joint, for example) and fluid (usually seen in the knees and ankles).

As the condition advances, the affected joint may become painful with even minimal movement, as well as when it is

CASE HISTORY

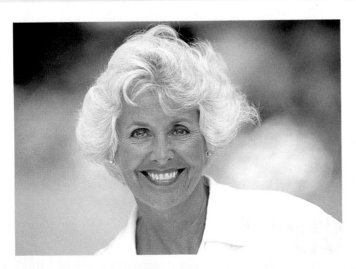

Catherine suffers from osteoarthritis, but it was years before a diagnosis was made:

"I have always made clothes and done a lot of sewing and upholstery in the house. I remember in my late forties my fingers seemed to be less nimble than they used to be, and occasionally the index finger on my right hand would feel creaky and stiff. I didn't really think about it much – I was so busy with the

house, my husband's business and the children at the time.

"In my late fifties, however, I started having problems with my hip and lower back. I had always worn shoes with heels and I am told now that this has thrown my hips out of true. This has meant excessive wear on both my hip joints and the joints of the knee as well.

"In my sixties, I started having the occasional fall. A fall really shakes you. I saw my doctor and he confirmed that it was all down to osteoarthritis.

"I know that I have osteoarthritis in several of my joints. It doesn't stop me doing anything that I want to do, but I know that I must not get too tired and I find standing for long periods difficult, so I try to avoid that. If I have had a particularly energetic day, I simply rest the next day and that seems to help. I think I'm lucky in that my hands don't look horribly arthritic, and I can still sew a little sometimes."

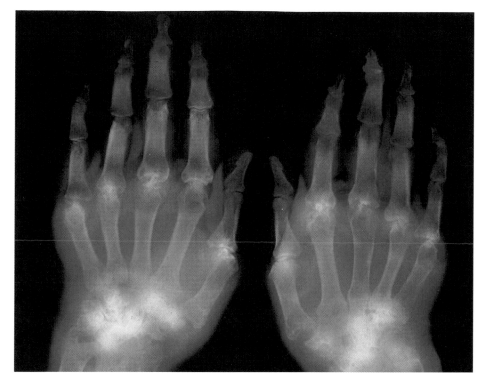

*An X-ray of arthritic
hands shows the
deformation of the first
joints of the fingers, that
is, those nearest the palm.
Most of the joints in
both hands show signs
of erosion. The joints
nearest the fingernails
are also frequently
affected by osteoarthritis.*

at rest and during the night. Osteoarthritis may also change the shape or size of bones. Outgrowths may form, and joints may take on a knobbled appearance.

Generally, stiffness of the joints is confined to a local area and lasts for only a short period of time, although there may also be some tenderness in the area of the affected joint.

Which joints are affected?

The joints most commonly affected by osteoarthritis are:
• The hands, particularly the joints of the fingers. Although men may be affected, osteoarthritis of the hands is 10 times more common in women.
• The knees, where you may experience pain and tenderness.
• The hips, in which case you may experience pain in the groin or inner thigh, and referred pain in the buttocks or the knee. You may find that movement of the hip becomes limited, particularly the rotating movement. Osteoarthritis of the hip affects men and women in equal numbers.
• The feet, especially the big toe.
• The spine, most commonly the lower back, but the vertebrae of the neck may also be affected, often referred to as spondylosis.

If you suspect that you have osteoarthritis, and in particular if a parent suffered from the condition, it is important to consult your doctor so that a firm diagnosis may be made. Doctors usually make a diagnosis based on a physical examination and by taking your medical history, along with an account of your symptoms. X-rays are used to confirm the diagnosis. The sooner a diagnosis is made, the better your chances of retaining mobility and controlling pain.

Rheumatoid arthritis

Rheumatoid arthritis is the commonest form of arthritis after osteoarthritis. It affects two to three times more women than men and usually starts between the ages of 25 and 50. Rheumatoid arthritis, unlike the wear-and-tear disorder of osteoarthritis, is an inflammatory disease of the immune system that affects the joints and other tissues.

The cartilage covering the head of the femur has been severely eaten away; only patches of healthy, smooth cartilage remain.

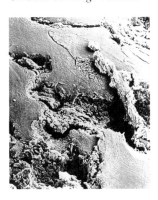

The primary symptoms of rheumatoid arthritis are joint pain and stiffness. Other symptoms include swelling in the joints, lack of appetite, low-grade fever, extreme fatigue and an overall feeling of being unwell. In addition, there may be nodules under the skin around the elbows and on the fingers.

In rheumatoid arthritis, inflammation starts in the synovial membrane lining the joints; this in turn leads to swelling or effusion in the joint space and damage to the bone (erosion). There may also be inflammation of the tendons, known as tenosynovitis, which makes the sufferer feel ill and tired.

The cause of rheumatoid arthritis is not known. It is much more distressing and troublesome than osteoarthritis both in the short and long term. It can strike at any age, including childhood, but it starts most frequently in youth or middle age. Rheumatoid arthritis affects people of all races, living in all climatic conditions, but the disease is more severe in the countries of northern Europe than in other parts of the world.

People who contract rheumatoid arthritis may have a single acute attack that persists for several months or longer, but which eventually clears up and never reappears. Or the disease may continue

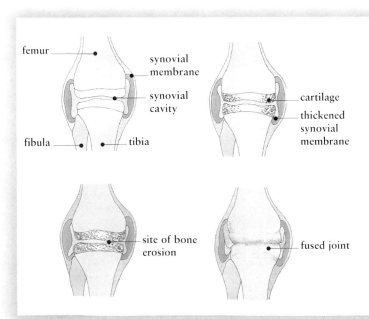

femur
synovial membrane
synovial cavity
fibula
tibia

cartilage
thickened synovial membrane

site of bone erosion

fused joint

RHEUMATOID ARTHRITIS

In a healthy knee joint (top, far left), the bones are covered by cartilage and the joint is lubricated by synovial fluid. In rheumatoid arthritis the cartilage thins and the synovial membrane becomes swollen and inflamed (top, left). As the condition progresses, the inflammation damages the cartilage (bottom, far left). In severe cases the cartilage becomes so thin that the bones are damaged and may even fuse together (bottom, left).

for the rest of their lives, when it is termed chronic. Only in a minority of cases does the disease persist to the point of becoming severely crippling.

Rheumatoid arthritis causes a deformity of the hands, whereby the fingers slant away from the thumb. This form of arthritis usually but not invariably affects both sides of the body symmetrically. Rheumatoid arthritis can affect the jaw occasionally and, rarely, the neck.

Find out more

Rheumatoid arthritis   *22–23*
What causes arthritis?   *30–37*

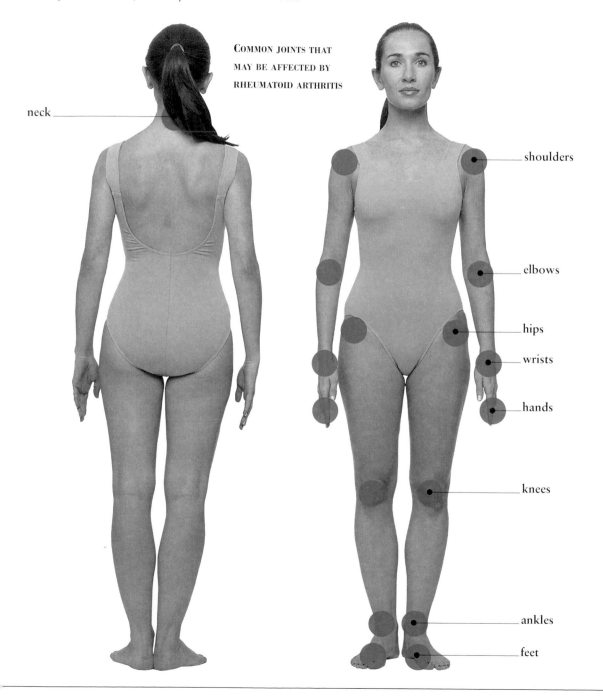

COMMON JOINTS THAT
MAY BE AFFECTED BY
RHEUMATOID ARTHRITIS

neck

shoulders

elbows

hips

wrists

hands

knees

ankles

feet

Rheumatoid arthritis

Rheumatoid arthritis and other forms of inflammatory arthritis are systemic diseases affecting the whole body, although the joints usually are the most affected. Other areas affected include the eyes, glands, mouth and blood vessels. In severe cases it can cause permanent damage to body tissue and the cartilage of the joints, and eventually deform and even destroy joints.

In some people, only one or two joints are affected. In others, the disease is widespread and very active. About 30 per cent of people who contract rheumatoid arthritis appear to recover completely within a few years. About 65 per cent continue to suffer pains in their joints, swellings and sudden flare-ups, while around 5 per cent become severely affected and extensively disabled.

If you develop painful, swollen joints, you should consult your doctor without delay. Confirmation of diagnosis is made by X-rays and blood tests that can detect the presence of inflammation. Your doctor may refer you to a consultant rheumatologist.

There is no need to respond to a diagnosis of rheumatoid arthritis with despair. Even in those people who have

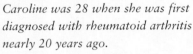

CASE HISTORY

Caroline was 28 when she was first diagnosed with rheumatoid arthritis nearly 20 years ago.

"I had noticed for quite some time that whenever I played tennis or went rowing, some of my joints would really hurt. It's hard to describe how painful it can be – and how mysteriously it seems to stop and start. I know that if I get upset it can get worse but it isn't always stress that triggers it. Sometimes it comes for no apparent reason.

"When I was first told by the doctor what the problem was, I thought it was effectively the end of my life. I could see myself crippled, in a wheelchair, unable to do anything for myself. I thought that I would be unable to have children – and that basically life would not be worth living.

"It has not been as bad as I thought it would be. I have given up tennis and rowing now – but I am still able to swim when the disease is not too acute. And I have two wonderful children. It was difficult while I was pregnant because all my joints were under a far greater strain than they had ever been before. And I was unable to take some of the drugs that I had been taking before I was pregnant.

"There have been times when I really have been completely incapacitated – and in a sense at those times my worst fears have been realized. The pain would sometimes be nearly unbearable. I was taking all the drugs prescribed by the consultant and I sometimes go to an aromatherapist, which does give some relief. I've tried other complementary therapies but none of them seem to work for me as well as aromatherapy.

"My big fear now is not so much for myself but for my two daughters. They are at some risk because of the genetic factor – and I cannot bear to think of either of them developing this illness."

severe rheumatoid arthritis, some find that they get better for no apparent reason. A sufferer may experience long periods of time with no symptoms. Absence of symptoms, or remission, can last days, months or even years.

Doctors use the following criteria to establish a positive diagnosis:
• The presence of arthritis for longer than six weeks
• Prolonged morning stiffness in the joints
• Presence of characteristic nodules under the skin
• Joint erosions seen on X-ray
• Positive blood tests of an antibody known as rheumatoid factor. However, 25 per cent of people with rheumatoid arthritis never develop this factor and some people who have the factor do not have rheumatoid arthritis.

Juvenile arthritis

Also known as Still's disease, arthritis affects one in 1,000 children every year. The majority of children with arthritis have what is known as acute reactive arthritis following a viral or bacterial infection. This type usually clears up within a few weeks or months.

Juvenile rheumatoid arthritis (JRA) is the most common type of persistent arthritis, lasting for months or years. There are three main forms of JRA.

Pauciarticular JRA

This is defined by the involvement of fewer than four joints at the start of the illness. It may start as a swollen knee or ankle which appears without injury or explanation. There may be no associated pain. This form is often very mild and can be treated with mild non-steroidal anti-inflammatory drugs.

Pauciarticular JRA can cause two important problems. The child may develop inflammation of the eye, which can, if left untreated, lead to scarring of the lens and permanent visual damage, even blindness. As the eye disease is more common in children who test positive for antinuclear antibodies (ANA), these children need to be examined by an eye specialist every three months. All other children with JRA need an eye examination every six months.

The second complication with pauciarticular JRA is that it may cause the bones in the legs to grow at different rates so that one leg is longer than the other, causing the child to limp. Limping damages the knee and the hip, leading to premature arthritis from "wearing out" the joints by the time the child reaches adulthood. This development should be prevented if at all possible.

Polyarticular JRA

This type of arthritis involves four or more joints from the start of the disease. It also usually worsens over time, but it can be treated successfully with non-steroidal anti-inflammatory drugs and, in severe cases, with gold shots or drugs such as sulphasalazine or methotrexate.

Systemic onset JRA

This more severe and more troublesome form of JRA starts with a high fever and a rash. The fever is usually high once or twice each day and then returns to normal. This type of JRA can affect the internal organs.

With prompt and appropriate treatment most children recover from JRA over time. Even children with severe cases should, if properly treated, manage to avoid becoming wheelchair-bound.

Find out more

Drug therapy   110–115

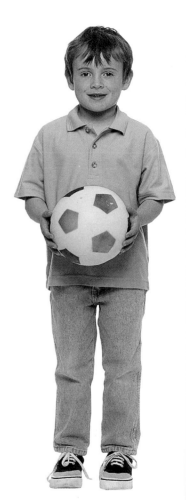

Because arthritis is often considered an illness of older people, there may be a delay in diagnosing arthritis in a child. But prompt diagnosis is important in the successful treatment of the condition.

Gout

Unlike many other forms of arthritis, gout affects more men than women. It most commonly affects the joint of the big toe. Gout is essentially the result of a defect in the body's internal chemistry – it is caused by uric acid crystals in the joints.

Uric acid is formed by the breakdown of chemicals called purines which derive from the genetic material of cells. It is normally excreted in the urine. If an excess of uric acid is produced, it accumulates and forms tiny crystals in the joints and elsewhere. If the crystals enter the joint space, they cause inflammation, swelling and severe pain. This is the condition known as gout.

Gout most commonly affects the big toe, but it may affect other joints: the ankles, knees, hands, wrists and elbows.

It can also affect the soft flesh of the ears, hands and feet, where uric acid may crystalize in the form of small hard white lumps called tophi.

The affected joint starts to ache, then quickly becomes swollen, red, very warm and extremely painful. The attack usually lasts for a few days, then dies down, and the joint gradually returns to normal.

Gout affects four times as many men as women. When gout affects women, it usually does so after the menopause when women have less natural protection against the disease. Gout is a controllable (although not curable) disease, but if left untreated, it can cause crippling arthritis, raised blood pressure and kidney damage, which may eventually prove fatal.

Some people are more susceptible to gout than others. In some people metabolism naturally handles uric acid slowly. Other triggers include infections, injury, antibiotics, diuretics (water tablets), aspirin and crash diets. Contrary to popular belief, food and drink intake play only a small role in gout.

Gout can be extremely painful and should always be taken seriously, despite its reputation for being the "disease of kings". It is important that an accurate diagnosis is made: although its symptoms may mimic other kinds of arthritis, the treatment for gout is specific.

Treatment for gout

There are three approaches to treatment. The first is caring for the pain. The second is treatment for the inflammation

HOW GOUT DEVELOPS

If the body produces too much uric acid, or fails to excrete it, excess acid is stored around the joints in the form of crystals. These deposits, called tophi, can be felt through the skin as small, hard lumps and may cause inflammation and swelling.

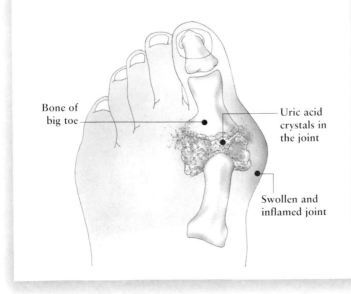

Bone of big toe

Uric acid crystals in the joint

Swollen and inflamed joint

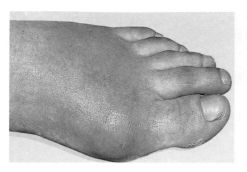

TELLTALE SIGNS

The inflamed, reddened area around the base of the big toe (left) is typical of gout. The inflammation is caused by crystals of uric acid in the fluid-filled spaces around a joint, typically in the toe joint.

with a course of anti-inflammatory drugs. You are advised to take plenty of rest, to increase your fluid intake, especially of water, and to greatly cut down on red meats and alcohol. The third treatment involves a combination of drugs, which you will have to take for the rest of your life. The first drug increases the excretion of uric acid via the kidneys (which necessitates, of course, an increased intake of fluids) and the second drug reduces the amount of acid produced by the body in the first place.

You may also be advised to limit your intake of foods high in purines, chemicals which can increase the amount of uric acid in the blood. Purine-rich foods include shellfish, oily fish and dried beans.

It is most important to take no painkillers if you suspect you have gout, except those prescribed by your doctor. Aspirin, for example, can actually slow the excretion of uric acid from the body, thereby aggravating the disease.

Pseudo gout

This is a form of arthritis caused by deposits of calcium crystals – rather than the uric acid crystals of gout – in the joints of the body. Pseudo gout refers to the gout-like attacks of joint inflammation that occur in many people suffering from this condition. The calcium-containing crystal deposits that are found in the cartilage of the joints may be visible on X-rays taken of the affected joint.

Pseudo gout is caused by deposits of crystals composed of calcium and pyrophosphate in the tissues of the body, especially the cartilage. It is believed that an accumulation of pyrophosphate in the cartilage promotes the formation of the crystals. Pyrophosphate is a type of acid produced by the joint tissues. In most cases, the crystals form without specific reason. Pseudo gout tends to run in families, as does true gout.

Acute attacks of pseudo gout often occur in the knee joints and can incapacitate the sufferer for weeks. Pseudo gout is not as serious (nor as painful) as gout and is harmless unless the crystals become dislodged. If this happens, they can set up inflammation in the joint. This is often treated by anti-inflammatory drugs or by drawing off the fluid containing the crystals with a syringe. Only if treatment is neglected is pseudo gout likely to cause long-term damage and pain.

Pseudo gout, like gout, is controllable but not curable. It is crucial that a correct diagnosis is made to avoid confusion with gout.

Excessive consumption of rich foods, such as red meat and alcoholic drinks, including red wine and port, possible triggers for gout.

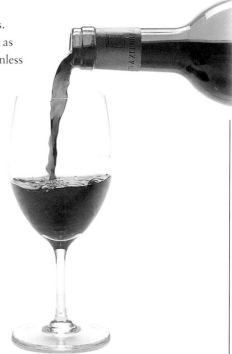

Other types of arthritis

*T*he less common forms of arthritic conditions include ankylosing spondylitis, lupus, psoriatic arthritis, infectious arthritis, septic arthritis, Sjögren's syndrome, fibromyalgia and polymyalgia rheumatica. There are also a number of rheumatic syndromes associated with HIV infection.

In some inflammatory forms of arthritis, the rheumatoid antibody – the marker for rheumatoid arthritis – is not found in the blood serum. These forms are known collectively as seronegative arthritis, and include ankylosing spondylitis, Reiter's disease, psoriatic arthritis and colitic arthritis, in which arthritis follows an infection.

Ankylosing spondylitis, which affects one person in 1,000, is a painful, progressive disease of the vertebrae of the spine. As a result of the inflammation,

scar tissue forms in the space between the vertebrae, making the joints stiff. This tissue may turn to bone so that when the inflammation dies down, it leaves bony deposits on the rims of the vertebrae. Bone grows from the sides of the affected vertebrae and may fuse together. If untreated this can cause severe deformity of the spine with the sufferer bent forward, hardly able to look up.

Ankylosing spondylitis affects many more men than women. Young men may develop the disease between the ages

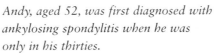

CASE HISTORY

Andy, aged 52, was first diagnosed with ankylosing spondylitis when he was only in his thirties.

"I used to play golf to competition standard. I took up squash, too, which I really enjoyed, and played several times a week. However, with time I was finding it more and more difficult to keep up my standard at squash. I had already given up golf, as my swing just wasn't up to it.

"A colleague had been diagnosed with ankylosing spondylitis, and he thought that I probably had it, too. I never was registered with a doctor and I didn't want to be told that there was something wrong with my back. I just wanted to go on playing. I found that

I had to book squash matches for the afternoon or evening, so that I could get myself limbered up. My back was always worse in the morning, I noticed.

"By my late forties, I just could not play any more, and I found that far from a good game of squash giving me the mobility that it had used to, it now made my back worse, so that I really suffered the next day.

"A couple of years ago, I went to see a chiropractor and he told me that all the vertebrae of my spine were fused together. Since that had already happened, the treatment he gave me didn't help all that much. What really helps is walking at a steady pace for several miles and regular heat treatments with massage. Nothing too strenuous!"

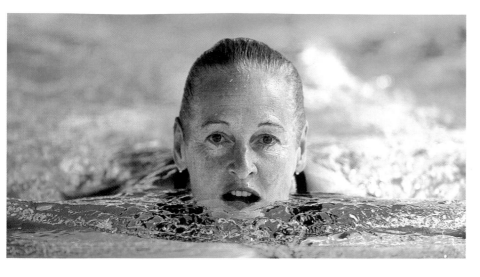

Swimming is an excellent non-weight bearing exercise that improves mobility in an arthritis sufferer. However, people with arthritis do not need to avoid all non-impact activities: brisk walking and running are both fine.

of 17 and 27, typically in their early twenties. There is a strong genetic factor linked to a tissues type called HLA 827. However, not all those who carry the gene develop the full-blown disease.

Symptoms

Ankylosing spondylitis starts with persistent back pain and early-morning stiffness that tends to become less with movement during the day. Symptoms may also include chronic fatigue and weight loss. There may be pain in the chest and ribs, making it difficult to breathe. Pain in the buttocks and the backs of the thighs, swollen ankles and tender heel bones may result.

The condition should be treated promptly, to avoid locking of the spine. Blood tests and X-rays are used to make a definitive diagnosis.

A relatively rare complication is iritis or uveitis, characterized by red, painful eyes. Go to hospital without delay if this happens to prevent permanent damage.

Treatment

There is no cure for ankylosing spondylitis, although you can slow the condition's advance by keeping mobile, and gain relief from pain through the application of heat. Hot baths, hot water bottles or an electric blanket, together with a firm bed, will prove helpful. Regular exercise, as advised by a physiotherapist, is important, so that even if fusion of the vertebrae takes place, the back fuses straight, rather than curved.

When you are working at a desk, change your position frequently so that you are not holding your spine in one fixed position for long periods.

FUSED BONES

As ankylosing spondylitis progresses, the joints of the spinal column become fused together into one continuous bone, producing a rigid spine. At the same time the discs and ligaments harden, further restricting mobility. At this stage, the condition may also be referred to as "bamboo spine".

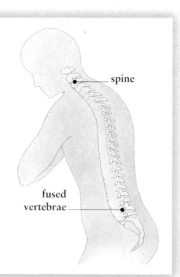

spine

fused vertebrae

Other types of arthritis

Systemic lupus erythematosus

Often known as lupus or SLE, this disease is a systemic auto-immune disorder producing a chronic inflammatory disease affecting all the organs of the body. Some three or four people in 100,000 suffer with this disease, which is more common in Afro-Caribbeans and some Asian populations than in Caucasians. Systemic lupus erythematosus is nine times more common in women than men.

In lupus, the immune system attacks the body's healthy tissues. This causes problems in all the systems of the body. Symptoms may include fever, malaise, weight loss, skin rashes, joint pain, breathing problems, kidney damage and gastrointestinal disorders, in addition to psychological symptoms.

Many drugs used to treat lupus suppress the function of the immune system, exposing the patient to increased risk of infection. Lupus can be caused by an infection or virus, by exposure to sunlight or by certain drugs.

Psoriatic arthritis

Arthritis can be associated with psoriasis. Psoriatic arthritis is an inflammation of the joints in people who already have psoriasis or who may develop psoriasis in the future. Psoriasis is a disease causing scaly, flaking skin and nails, which affects about one in 50 of the population. Of those with psoriasis, about one in 10 will develop the associated arthritis. The condition can affect people of all ages, and women and men are affected in equal numbers.

Painful inflammation at the bony sites where ligaments and tendons are attached, for example at the heels, is also associated with psoriatic arthritis.

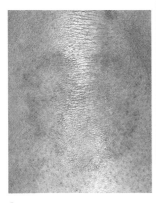

Lupus may cause a blotchy red rash on the skin. The rash, like the condition itself, subsides and then recurs.

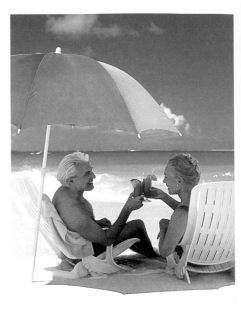

The lupus rash can be triggered by exposure to sunlight. Use a sunscreen with an SPF of 15 or more, wear a brimmed hat and stay in the shade as much as possible, especially during the hottest parts of the day.

Infectious arthritis

Arthritis may be triggered by varoius viral infections, notably rubella (German measles). This form of arthritis is usually curable provided that it is treated promptly. Without treatment, however, infectious arthritis can lead to serious damage to the joints and it may spread to other parts of the body.

Most types of infectious arthritis are caused by bacteria, but they can also be caused by viruses, such as infectious hepatitis, mumps and glandular fever. Fungal arthritis is less common.

Septic arthritis

Triggered by a penetrating injury or other infection, such as tuberculosis or gonorrhoea, septic arthritis means the joint becomes infected. There may be an earlier history of an infected lesion such as an ingrown toenail, boil or an ulcerating nodule. Septic arthritis causes a joint to be hot and painful and disproportionally inflamed compared with other joints. Treatment is by aspiration, or drainage and antibiotics.

Sjögren's syndrome

In this disorder chronic arthritis is accompanied by dry eyes and dry mouth. Other symptoms include irritation, a gritty feeling or painful burning in the eyes. The eyelids may stick together. Food is difficult to chew and swallow because it sticks in the throat. The voice may be thin and reedy and the teeth may start to degenerate. Treatment is usually the same as for rheumatoid arthritis.

Fibromyalgia

Also known as fibrositis, fibromyalgia is a condition that causes widespread aching, stiffness and fatigue. It originates in the muscles and soft tissues of the body. People with this condition are found to have multiple tender points in specific muscle areas. Symptoms include aching and stiffness around the neck, shoulders, upper back, lower back and hip areas. There may also be pain in the chest and knees, sleep disturbance, irritable bowel syndrome and migraine.

Fibromyalgia does not respond to aspirin or paracetamol, and stronger analgesics may be ineffective. Hot baths, relaxation exercises and massage can all bring relief. Swimming in warm water and exercises to improve posture and tone the muscles are also recommended.

Polymyalgia rheumatica

Polymyalgia rheumatica is a disorder typically suffered by people over the age of 50. The condition causes severe stiffness and aching in the muscles of the neck, shoulder and hip areas. Other symptoms include inflammation of the arteries, which can cause blindness, fatigue, weight loss, low fever and depression. It occurs twice as often in women as in men. Treatment involves corticosteroids.

Find out more

Alexander technique	*74–77*
Drug therapy	*110–115*
Exercise	*148–151*

CASE HISTORY

Nicola, aged 36, suffers from lupus.

"I already had severe arthritis and was finding life difficult – even washing and dressing myself had become a problem. Then the rash appeared. Lupus was diagnosed several months later. The disease has affected my brain so that I cannot remember things. I have to carry a card with my name and address on it.

"The chemotherapy treatment is horrible – I have to have it to suppress the immune system to prevent it attacking *my body. But after the chemo, I get all sorts of unpleasant infections like mouth ulcers and so on.*

"I also have to have kidney dialysis, while I'm waiting for a transplant. I get all sorts of side-effects from the drugs, but I have to have them. When the illness flares up, as it does from time to time, I'm so exhausted that I can't do anything except stay in bed and rest."

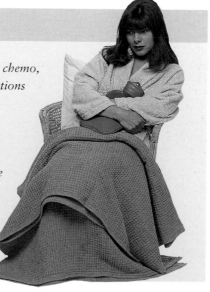

What causes arthritis?

Arthritis, in its many forms, has varied and complex causes. Increasing age is the primary factor in some forms of the disease; in others a breakdown in the body's chemistry is responsible; and in some arthritic conditions a malfunction of the immune system may be to blame.

Cycling is excellent for improving cardiovascular fitness and boosting the metabolism, thereby aiding weight loss. Note that strenuous cycling can put stress on the knees.

Research is currently under way into the causes of arthritis, which include understanding how the immune system works and what goes wrong in many types of arthritis. The stages and mechanisms of the auto-immune reaction, in which the body's own tissues are attacked by antibodies, are becoming clear and they offer hope for the development of new treatments.

Most diseases become worse with increasing age – there are few that we "grow out of". Therefore, while age may not be a cause of the majority of arthritic conditions, the ageing process naturally plays its part in accelerating the disease and weakening the body's immune and defence mechanisms, thereby rendering the body less able to fight the disease. In addition, as we age, the metabolism slows, predisposing the body to weight gain. This can affect the development and progression of arthritis.

Some risk factors are within your own control – you can lose weight, you can stop smoking and you can generally improve your lifestyle with a view to alleviating your arthritis.

Too much weight

People who are carrying too much body weight are, clearly, putting excessive strain on all their body's systems. The joints of the musculo-skeletal system are no exception: they have to work harder if you are overweight. What is normally a degenerative or wear and tear disease in people of average weight becomes a more serious risk to health in obese people.

The delicate mechanisms of the joints, particularly the weight-bearing joints, such as the hips, knees and ankles are stretched to the limit. For example, the vertebrae of the spine will become compressed. The cartilage surrounding the ends of bone becomes less springy. The muscles and joints require more

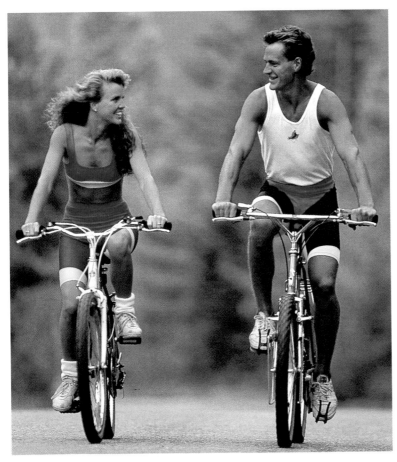

oxygen – but the overweight body with an impaired cardiovascular system cannot produce sufficient oxygen quickly enough to meet the demand. Because of the way joints work, the strain on crucial parts of the joint can be magnified four or five times, so a small weight loss can make a big difference to the strain on a weight-bearing joint.

Arthritis is significantly more common in overweight women – decreased mobility is nearly twice as frequent. Being overweight is clearly unhelpful to those suffering with osteoarthritis and it is recommended that sufferers should do their best to return to a normal weight for their height. Obesity is also a factor in other types of arthritis, since daily life is more exhausting if you are overweight.

How much is too much?

Traditional ways of deciding whether or not we are of a healthy weight, such as height/weight charts, are no longer regarded as a sufficiently accurate guideline of ideal weight. Nor do they take account of the proportion of fat to muscle in the body. Since muscle weighs more than fat, you may be heavier than someone of the same height, but actually fitter. Doctors today use the Body Mass Index (BMI) to ascertain whether your weight is in the normal range. This is explained in full on pages 116–117.

The heredity factor

Many types of arthritis can be seen to occur with greater frequency in some families than in others. However, this is not to say that arthritis is "inherited". The most one can say is that you may have inherited a genetic predisposition to that disease if your parents, grandparents, uncles and aunts have it.

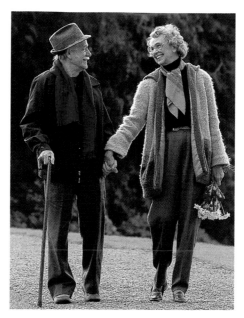

Find out more

What causes arthritis?   32–37
Physical therapies   116–121
Exercise   146–149

Osteoporosis, or brittle bones, may be aggrevated by other factors often found in arthritis sufferers. One way to help maintain bone density is to take a brisk walk of half an hour's duration at least three times a week – it will also help to keep your weight in the normal range.

AGE

Increasing age is a common cause of some types of arthritis and a determining factor in other types.

- *In osteoarthritis, the most common type of arthritis, nearly 70 per cent of people over the age of 70 have some arthritis visible on X-ray. This type is without doubt a "wear and tear" disease, a normal part of the ageing process.*
- *Age may be a factor in rheumatoid arthritis, but it is not a cause. The usual onset for rheumatoid arthritis is between the ages of 25 and 50.*
- *The development of gout is related to age, but not caused by age. An inbuilt metabolic disfunction may eventually lead to the formation of uric acid crystals, which are responsible for the characteristic pain of gout.*
- *Age plays a determining role in the development of ankylosing spondylitis without being a cause of the disease. The usual onset of this condition is between the ages of 17 and 27.*
- *Systemic lupus erythematosus, or lupus, usually affects women between the ages of 15 and 45 (the childbearing years), although the disease can, in significantly fewer numbers, affect younger and older women as well as men.*

What causes arthritis?

Scientists are still unable to say whether arthritis is inherited or not, but if several members of your family have suffered from the disease it is worth asking your doctor to test whether you are showing signs. Early diagnosis usually results in greater success in treatment.

The genetic factor

Is arthritis genetic? More than one gene has been implicated in the development of arthritis, notably rheumatoid arthritis. However, just because you have that gene does not necessarily mean that you will go on to develop the disease. Equally, some people who do not carry the gene may in fact develop the disease. There is a strong inherited tendency to develop some forms of osteoarthritis. Heredity is a major factor in ankylosing spondylitis.

Gene research

Researchers have found a specific sequence of nucleic acid, one of the building blocks of DNA (the body's genetic blueprint), that is a marker for

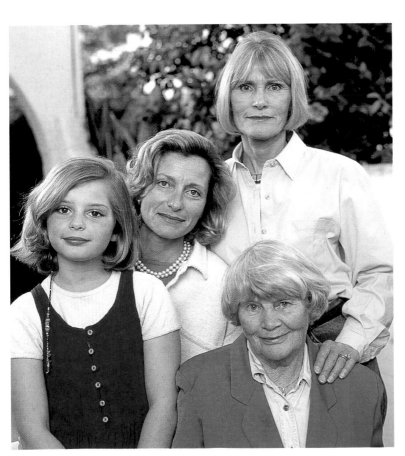

rheumatoid arthritis. People who inherit this sequence from both their father and mother are more likely to have a severe form of the disease, which could involve internal organs as well as joints. This type of research may lead in the future to genetic counselling, in order to help identify people at greater risk for developing more severe forms of arthritis or needing more intensive treatment.

The cause of arthritis and the search for the gene responsible is still a matter of concentrated scientific research. Genetic factors are known to play a role in predisposing people to rheumatoid arthritis, but scientists do not yet know about all the genes that are involved.

In September 1997 in the United States, the Arthritis Foundation, the National Institute of Arthritis, Musculoskeletal and Skin Diseases and the National Institute of Allergy and Infectious Diseases joined forces to support a national consortium of 12 research centres in the search for genes that determine susceptibility to rheumatoid arthritis. The group, the North American Rheumatoid Arthritis Consortium (NARAC), hopes to learn more about the genes that play a role in causing the disease.

It will be some years before the results of this study are known. For now, scientists believe rheumatoid arthritis may result from a combination of genetic factors that make a person susceptible to the disease and a certain environmental trigger, possibly an infectious agent such as a virus or bacterium.

The gender factor

Is arthritis more common in women than in men? Ankylosing spondylitis is one of the few forms of arthritis which appears more often in men than in women. Most other types, however, affect a much higher percentage of women than men.

In the USA nearly two-thirds of all people with the disease are women.
• Osteoarthritis affects 11.7 million women, which represents 74 per cent of all cases of the disease.
• Fibromyalgia affects 3.7 million people and seven times more women than men.
• Rheumatoid arthritis affects 1.5 million women, or 71 per cent of cases.
• Lupus affects 117,000 women, or 89 per cent of all cases.
• Juvenile rheumatoid arthritis affects 61,000 girls, which represents 86 per cent of all cases.

Autoimmunity

Many forms of arthritis, including rheumatoid arthritis and SLE, involve autoimmunity. Autoimmunity is the process when the body's immune system "makes a mistake" and starts to attack parts of the body. It is generally thought that this process is triggered by an infection, either bacterial or viral, which sets off the immune reaction, and which does not switch off in the normal way when the infection clears up. In most cases it is not certain exactly what the infection involved is.

Exercise and sport

In the normal scheme of things, exercise is beneficial, and most people would gain by doing more exercise. This said, there are certain types of exercise and sport that can aggravate arthritis if you are already predisposed to it and certain forms of exercise and sports that may actually cause the disease.

The stresses and strains that various ballet positions and techniques place on the joints of the body represent an intolerable burden and the joints suffer.

Contact sports frequently cause joint problems, cartilage problems and arthritis in later years. Football – which may lead to problems with the knees – is probably the best known example, but rugby football and other sports are harmful.
• The repetitive nature of some types of exercise may cause problems at any age.
• Many sports are hazardous simply because of their potential for trauma or injury. Any sport in which you might fall and break a bone, or suffer an injury requiring surgery may predispose you to later problems.
• The fact that many forms of exercise and sport are competitive puts the body in a state of tension, increases the potential for trauma and wear and tear. Sports that require an unnatural position to be held for some time while the body is in a state of tension are particularly hazardous. The knees and, in some people, hips are liable to suffer under such strain.

Exercise in moderation. Don't place too great a burden on your body. In particular, avoid sports that involve twisting and turning movements. If you do suffer aches and pains after sport or exercise, take this as a warning: your body is telling you that the strain is too much. Don't be tempted to ignore the warning and continue with the exercise. Take a few days out for rest and allow the body to recuperate. And, next time you play your favourite sport, or take any form of exercise, wear well-fitting padded footwear, be sure to warm up properly before you start, take care during exercising, stop as soon as you start to feel tired, and cool down properly.

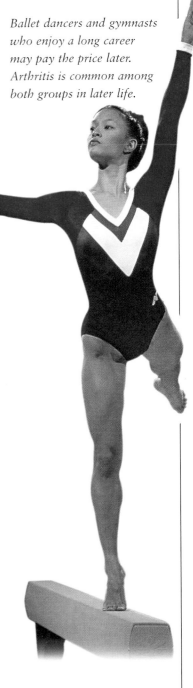

Ballet dancers and gymnasts who enjoy a long career may pay the price later. Arthritis is common among both groups in later life.

CHAPTER ONE

What causes arthritis?

Medication

Because some drugs can interact with others and some combinations of drugs can produce unwanted side-effects in the form of arthritis, it is essential that you check with your doctor before taking any medication. Your doctor should be aware of all the other drugs that you are taking so that he or she can check for possible interaction. This is especially important in gout, for example, because the very treatment that can relieve other types of arthritis – aspirin – can promote gout.

Arthritis drugs can react with certain medications prescribed for lowering blood pressure and with lithium (a psychotropic drug prescribed for manic depression. The rubella vaccination produces musculo-skeletal symptoms in 20 per cent of cases. These usually last for two to four weeks after the vaccination, but they may persist for several weeks, and, in rare instances, even months. Intravenous drug

The rubella (German measles) vaccine may produce short-lived arthritis, as does contracting rubella itself. If you have symptoms, tell your doctor if you have recently been immunized against, or contracted, German measles.

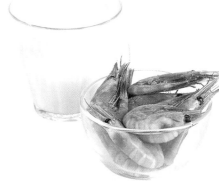

Many foods can set up an allergic reaction in susceptible individuals. Among the most common are dairy products, such as milk and cheese, wheat and wheat products, and shellfish.

users are at risk of developing septic arthritis.

When you receive a prescription, follow a few simple precautions.
• Check that the drug written down is the one the doctor told you he or she intended to prescribe.
• Ask your doctor if there are known side-effects with the drug, so that you have an idea what to expect.
• When you collect the drug at the pharmacy, check the label to be sure that what you have been given is what your doctor intended to prescribe.

Mistakes can and do happen: human error is part of everyday life.

Allergies

An allergic reaction is a damaging immune response of the body to a substance (especially a specific food, pollen, fur or dust) to which it has become hypersensitive.

Food allergies may play a role in some types of inflammatory arthritis. It is important that you ask your doctor to

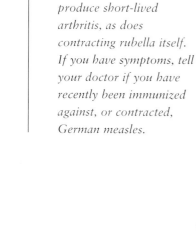

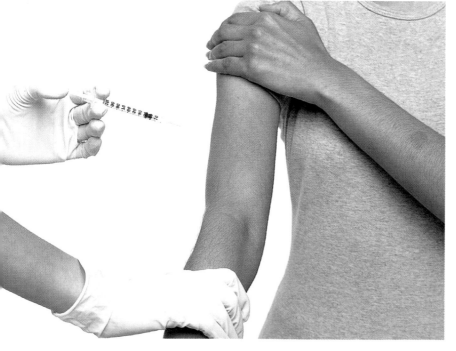

refer you for allergy investigations at a hospital if you are suffering arthritis pains without any other evidence of arthritis. An allergy may well be to blame.

No matter the disease or disorder, it is always important that a correct diagnosis is made as soon as possible, so that prompt and proper treatment can follow.

Trauma (injury)

Trauma is defined as any physical wound or injury. Arthritis sometimes develops after an injury that damages a joint, regardless of any genetic predisposition to the disease. The arthritis may develop many years after the trauma. This type of arthritis is known as secondary arthritis.

Find out more

Drug therapy	*110–115*
Diet	*142–147*

CASE HISTORY

Rosie, now in her late 30s, has been diagnosed as having secondary arthritis.

"When I was 14, I was out with our dog and she was running toward the road. I ran down a slope that was damp with dew. I was running as fast as I possibly could to catch her, but I slipped and my leg ended up beneath me. The pain was unimaginable. It turned out that I had broken both the main bones of my leg and sprained my knee.

"A few years later when I was 17, I was in Paris and I slipped on a couple of steps. I was wearing sandals that didn't stay on too well. My ankle was extremely painful but because I was on holiday I didn't go to the doctor. I managed to hobble around for a couple of days before I saw someone. I was taken to hospital without delay and put in plaster, and told to rest. It turned out that I had been walking on a broken right ankle for more than two days.

Some years later, when I was working in Hong Kong, by now I was 22, I slipped – again – and turned my ankle (the same one that I had broken in Paris). It was pretty painful but I didn't think too much about it. The next day, however, the ankle was extremely swollen, painful and immobile, so I went
 to the hospital for an X-ray. I'm told that the X-ray showed nothing.

"A few days later, I was still in pain so I went to my own doctor this time, and he referred me to an orthopaedic surgeon. He took fresh X-rays, which he examined with an eagle eye. He found that the ankle was fractured again, and, on top of that, a small piece of bone, which had apparently formed a spur as a result of the previous fracture, had now broken off and was floating around. The surgeon proposed to operate and remove the bone fragment and get me into plaster.

"I suppose it is not surprising after these injuries, plus the fact that I was actually walking on an injured joint more than once, that my right ankle is not as strong as the left one. I'm nearly 40 now, and the injured ankle sometimes swells up for no reason; it aches, especially in damp weather; and it is distinctly wobbly when I wear high heels. I know I've got arthritis in that ankle, and I do wish I'd been more sensible in my younger days!"

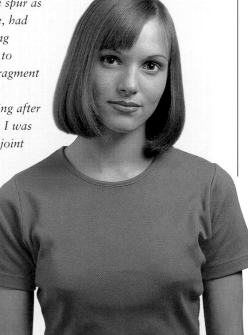

What causes arthritis?

Smoking

Cigarette smoking causes more than 100,000 premature deaths a year in the United Kingdom, 23,000 premature deaths in Australia and around 350,000 annually in the United States. Few smokers can claim ignorance of the medical hazards of smoking. While smoking is in decline in the developed world, it is on the increase in some developing countries.

Smoking is hazardous not only for the diseases that it actually causes, such as lung cancer, but also for the fact that virtually every disease and disorder is made worse by smoking. Arthritis is no exception. Tobacco contains toxic substances and smoking subverts up to about 15 per cent of the body's oxygen supply. This means that regeneration of damaged tissue takes longer and pain and fatigue are greater in arthritis sufferers who smoke than in those who do not.

Smoking and arthritis research

In September 1997, the *Annals of the Rheumatic Diseases* published a report stating that smoking increases the severity of rheumatoid arthritis. Researchers at the University of Iowa College of Medicine in the USA studied the severity of the disease in more than 300 patients. They concluded that smoking is a significant, modifiable risk factor that affects the severity of rheumatoid arthritis. Their study is the first to investigate the effect of smoking on arthritis sufferers.

Rheumatoid arthritis causes chronic inflammation and degeneration of the joints, typically those in the fingers, hands, feet, ankles, knees and shoulders. The condition is usually diagnosed by the presence of swollen joints, by X-rays that reveal erosion around the affected joints and by the presence of antibodies in the blood known as rheumatoid factor.

After adjusting for known risk factors of rheumatoid arthritis, such as age and gender, the University of Iowa team found that patients who had smoked in the past or were current smokers were more likely to have high levels of rheumatoid factor and were at an increased risk for bone erosion. Moreover, those sufferers who had smoked for more than 25 years had three times the rheumatoid factor and bone erosion risks of non-smokers.

The dangers

Smoking can cause abnormalities in the immune system of rheumatoid arthritis sufferers – in the lungs and other parts of the body. Smoking increases a person's white blood cell count and heavy smoking can cause abnormalities in immune system cells that may increase the risk of infection. Smoking compromises the activities of the immune system throughout the body and the authors of the study suggest that it may be more important in the initiation of erosive disease than in perpetuating the process.

Lifestyle

There are steps you can take to lessen your risk of developing arthritis or to alleviate it if you are already a sufferer.

Lessening the risks

1. Keep your weight within the normal range for your height. If you are not sure what this is, calculate your Body Mass Index (see pages 116–117).
2. Eat a healthy diet. Have five portions of fresh fruit or vegetables a day, eaten raw or lightly steamed to preserve their vitamin and mineral content. Eat foods rich in iron and calcium, and consider

supplements of fish oil, which are rich in the omega-3 essential fats known as EPA and DHA.

3. Always exercise and play sport in moderation, with some thought for the stresses on your musculo-skeletal system. Pay particular attention if your work places undue strain on your body.

4. Check out your medications with your doctor and with the pharmacy that supplies them.

5. If you believe that any of your joints are affected by arthritis, consult your doctor with a view toward beginning treatment as soon as possible. The sooner treatment starts, the greater your chances of retaining mobility

6. After injury, reduce the pain and stress on your joints by finding out which exercise and relaxation techniques work best for you. Appropriate exercise (see Chapter 3) can protect a joint against further damage. Remember that it is as harmful to under-use joints and muscles as it is to over-use them.

7. It helps to learn how to strike a balance between being able to relax and keeping as fit and active as possible. Relaxation classes help some people, as do other complementary therapies such as meditation, visualization, acupuncture and aromatherapy. The complementary therapies are described in more complete detail in Chapter 2.

Although fewer people overall are smoking, rates are still high among young people: for example, 20 per cent of young men are smokers, laying themselves open to later health problems, including arthritis.

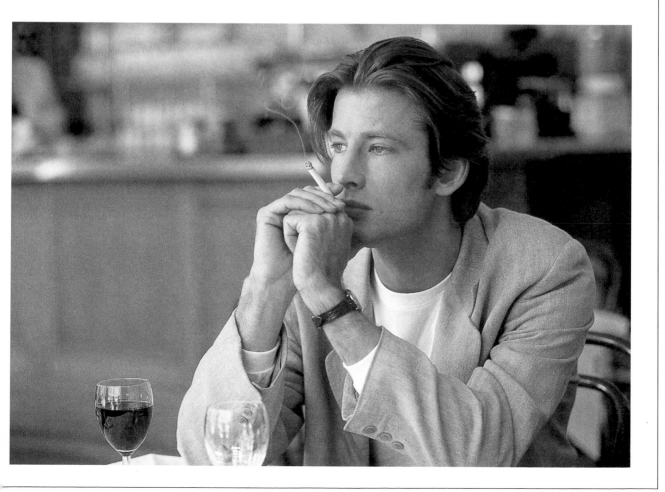

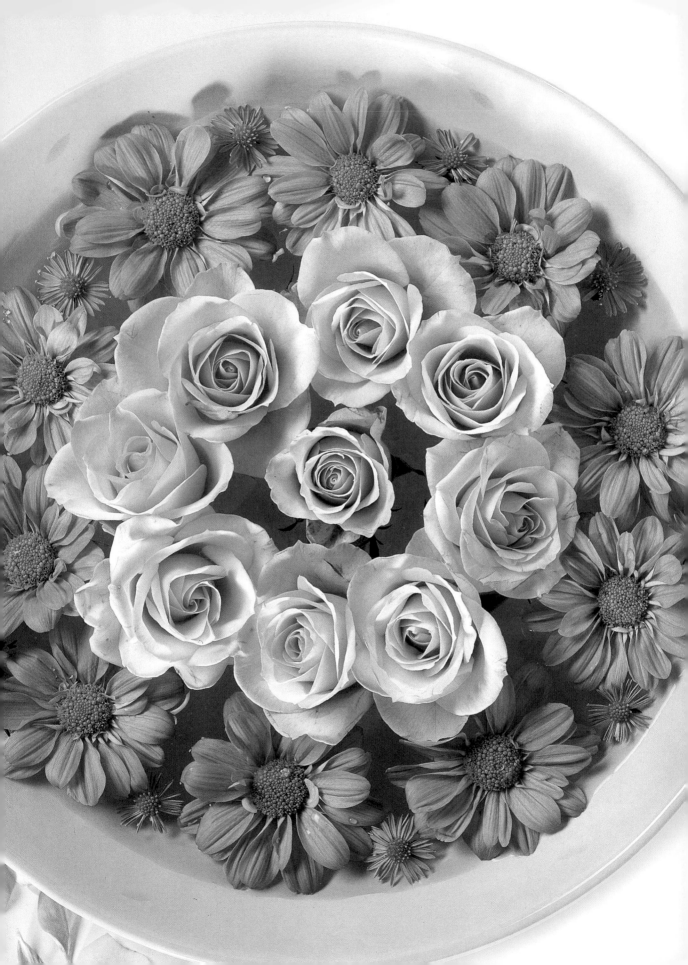

2

COMPLEMENTARY

TREATMENTS

Because arthritis is so common, much effort has been spent researching orthodox treatments to prevent or reverse the condition. So far, this has not been fully successful.

Orthodox drugs can do much to overcome the agonizing pain that arthritis in its various forms can cause, but they may cause serious side-effects. In addition, prescription drugs do not relieve the misery, resentment and bitterness often sustained by arthritis sufferers.

This is where complementary therapies can help. They provide gentle but effective adjuncts and alternatives to strong drugs, providing relief without side-effects. In fact, complementary therapies are often used by orthodox doctors.

Why choose complementary?

Complementary therapies are usually gentle, without the adverse reactions that can occur with conventional medicines. They are designed to work with the body, so knowing the medical history of the person being treated is important.

Many of the complementary therapies that have become popular in Western society over the past few decades have their roots in Eastern cultures, and they have been practised for hundreds of years. These include acupuncture, yoga and meditation. Others, such as the Alexander technique, osteopathy and chiropractic, are late arrivals and were developed in Western countries.

Although the terms "alternative" and "non-orthodox" may be used when referring to complementary therapies, they are misnomers. First of all, as any responsible complementary practitioner will tell you, complementary therapies should be used alongside conventional medical treatments – not as an alternative. Today, complementary therapies are recognized by many traditional Western practitioners, and some of them also practise complementary therapies.

Mainstream medicine and complementary therapies rely on different approaches for treatment. Conventional doctors try to cure or treat a condition that has already presented itself. According to them, arthritis is a condition that has no fully understood cause and no cure. Their aim is to treat the symptoms, and they often prescribe drugs – a mainstay of conventional medicine – to override the pain, inflammation and stiffness of arthritis. These drugs do not always make you feel better, nor improve your overall health.

Complementary therapies are holistic. They attempt to boost the body's own natural defences by treating the complete person, including his or her physical, mental, emotional and spiritual states. Because complementary treatments are holistic, they can enhance your general health and wellbeing as well as treat your arthritis.

Some of the therapies, including acupuncture, shiatsu and reflexology, are based on the idea of a "life force" that flows through the body. Illness can occur if the channels, or meridians, that allow the life force to travel through the body become blocked. By unblocking the channels the practitioner can help the body to return to good health.

Your choice

There is a huge variety of complementary therapies available to treat arthritis, and they take many forms (see pp.42–43). There are the medicinal therapies such as homeopathy and herbal medicine, and the physical therapies include massage and

Acupuncture needles stimulate points on the body's meridians to enhance the flow of qi, *the life force, through the body and restore health.*

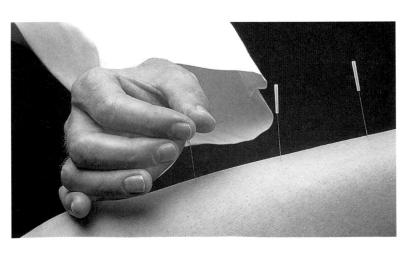

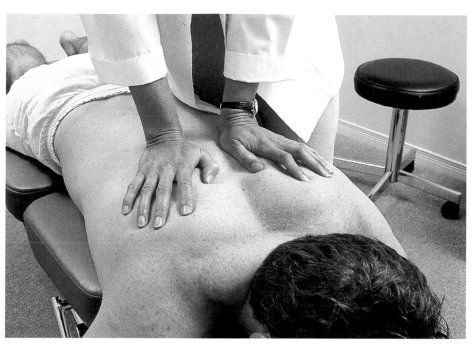

Find out more

*Acupuncture
and acupressure* 78–81
Chiropractic 92–93

*Chiropractors believe that
the body's innate ability
to heal itself stems from the
central nervous system.
If the spine is misaligned,
the body is unable to
restore balance to the
tissues and joints.*

the Alexander technique. In fact, there is such a wide range of therapies offered, that you can choose whether to do them by yourself at home, in a class or by regularly visiting a practitioner. Depending on the type and severity of your arthritis, you can choose a hands-on approach, as with massage, or a supervised diet and exercise programme. You can visit a spa for water treatment, or go for an ancient Eastern remedy such as acupuncture or shiatsu.

Complementary treatments demand some active input from you, the patient. By choosing a complementary therapy, you are putting yourself in control, taking responsibility for your own health. You will also be helping yourself to adopt a more positive, optimistic state of mind than before, and this in itself aids the healing process.

Consultations with complementary therapists usually take about an hour. The practitioner will ask all kinds of questions about yourself and your medical history, not just the arthritis. You will be treated as an individual, not as a case of arthritis.

Are there any disadvantages to choosing complementary approaches? Yes – they may not work as quickly as conventional medicine, and they require that added effort on your part.

AVAILABLE THERAPIES

Acupressure and acupuncture
Alexander technique
Aromatherapy
Biofeedback
Chiropractic
Colour therapy
Dance therapy
Herbal medicine
Homeopathy
Hydrotherapy
Massage

Meditation
Naturopathy
Osteopathy
Psychotherapy and counselling
Reflexology
Relaxation
Self-hypnosis
Shiatsu
T'ai chi
Visualization
Yoga

Choosing a complementary therapy

Non-orthodox medicine is becoming ever more popular for dealing with chronic diseases such as arthritis. Disappointment with conventional treatments offered by standard medicine often leads sufferers towards unusual therapies that they might never have considered when well._

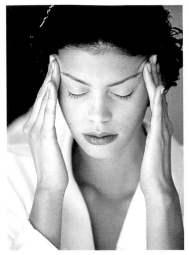

Learning simple techniques to relieve pain can increase your confidence in your ability to control your condition.

Having decided that you might like to try a complementary therapy, where do you start when there are so many different therapies on offer? And how do you discover whether they will work? Medical doctors and consultants have to go through rigorous training programmes, but the same standards do not apply to all complementary medicine. Things are improving, but it is still the case that anybody can legally set up as alternative practitioner without having been through a training course. Try finding a registered therapist who, by law, must carry a license supplied by his professional council.

Many general practitioners will refer you to an alternative therapist, and some alternative therapies are now included in private health insurance coverage – provided that they have the backing of a qualified doctor.

When evaluating a particular therapy or regime, you would be wise to ask yourself such questions as:

• Would I mind being almost completely undressed while being massaged?
• Could I stick to an extremely limited dietary regime?
• Could I tolerate having acupuncture needles stuck into me?
• Do I like the idea of talking the whole experience of the illness through with a psychotherapist?
• Would I have the time and patience to carry out a daily meditation programme?
• How far am I prepared to alter or modify my lifestyle?

Another critical yardstick is how much time you are prepared to give to a particular therapy and how you can build it into your life.

You should also consider what costs you can afford to pay.

Your degree of mobility might also affect your choice of treatment.

Precautions

Whatever you decide, don't just come off your pain-killing medication because you are taking another approach. Control of pain and inflammation is important, and in most cases, non-orthodox treatments will work well in conjunction with medical drugs. There may be exceptions, however, as for some homeopathic or herbal remedies, so never embark on these treatments without first consulting your conventional doctor. You should also tell your homeopath or herbalist what drugs you are taking.

Any reputable complementary therapist should be prepared to talk with your doctor if necessary; in fact, a therapist may well recommend that you consult your general practitioner before you start a course of complementary treatment. Be wary of any complementary therapist who talks disparagingly about conventional medicine.

Mind and body

A final question to ask yourself is: do I want the complementary therapy to work directly on the arthritis, or to help me cope with the anxiety, depression and stress that seem to come with the condition? Many people who suffer from arthritis become depressed to some degree and it is perhaps inevitable that you will feel bitter at times about having an incurable condition.

It is increasingly being accepted that, with all major diseases, thought processes affect physical processes. Certain alternative regimes such as visualization and meditation will help replace negative thoughts with positive thoughts, and soothe you so that the pain abates – but, helpful as they are, such therapies cannot directly ease the arthritis.

By contrast, a strict dietary regime that cuts out all acid-forming substances such as alcohol, cigarettes, caffeine and white sugar, and replaces them with alkaline-forming foods such as fresh vegetables and pulses, can have a direct effect on the joints. However, you may consider such a diet difficult or impossible to follow.

Manipulative therapies, such as osteopathy and chiropractic, can ease and, to some extent, correct deformed, twisted joints. Acupuncture also purports to work directly on the condition. A therapy such as the Alexander technique uses both mental and physical means to bring about dramatic health improvement, particularly where posture is affected by the illness. The same is true of yoga. But, in order to work, such therapies need a commitment and constant practice.

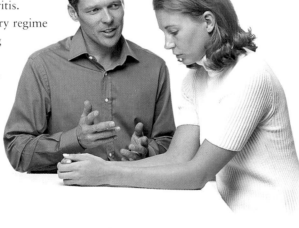

Find out more

*Why choose
complementary?* *40–41*
Choosing a practitioner 106–107

It is worth taking time to find the therapy that suits you best and a practitioner with whom you feel comfortable. Your relationship with your therapist becomes an integral part of the healing process.

POINTS TO CONSIDER

The choice of complementary therapies is huge – and it's up to you to decide. Bear in mind these important factors:
- *There is no proven cure for arthritis – you should be suspicious of any complementary practitioner who assures you that there is.*
- *All complementary therapies demand input from you. Your involvement may be very time-consuming.*

- *Ensure that your therapist has taken an accredited course of training. You may want to contact the relevant professional body to confirm the therapist's qualifications.*
- *Before signing up for an expensive regime, ask to be put in touch with satisfied clients.*
- *Check with your doctor before starting any non-orthodox therapy.*

Yoga

Yoga was developed over 2,000 years ago as a means of aiding meditation and to enable spiritual energy to travel through the body. At its heart lies the notion of gaining control – of the body, mind and spirit – by gentle, effective means.

This ancient discipline brings the body's various systems into harmony while increasing suppleness and improving posture. The word *yoga* is Sanskrit for "union" and has two distinct but related aspects: *pranayama*, or breathing, and the *asanas*, or postures. Yoga remained a strictly Eastern discipline, practised almost entirely by men as a means of gaining spiritual enlightenment, until after the First World War, when it began to gain some popularity in the West as part of the then new "nature cure". Yoga postures were practised at spas and sanatoriums all over Europe, although the discipline continued to be considered "cranky" by the average Westerner.

After the Second World War, however, yoga was taken up enthusiastically as a keep-fit regime with a bit of undemanding spirituality thrown in. Yoga teacher Richard Hittleman, and later Lyn Marshall, introduced yoga to a mass audience in the United Kingdom through their highly popular television programmes during the 1960s and 1970s.

Nowadays, you can find yoga classes at almost every local keep-fit centre, and there are countless books and videos available on the subject, as well as retreats and ashrams offering residential courses.

Yoga is often jokingly called "the ancient art of tying yourself up in knots"; so what does it have to do with arthritis and how can it benefit the arthritis sufferer? You would have to be at almost international gymnast standard to attain some of the postures, and even the easiest asanas are beyond most arthritis sufferers.

Yoga therapy

The answer lies in a specially adapted form of yoga known as yoga therapy. This is gentler and easier than standard yoga, and takes into account the stiffness and immobility of arthritic joints. Yoga therapy for arthritis has been available for more than 40 years in the West, but only at specialized alternative centres.

For the past few years, however, the Yoga Biomedical Trust, founded by Dr Robin Munro, has been researching and developing yoga for use by people with chronic or serious complaints that continue to baffle the medical profession. It was after Dr Munro's own asthma was cured by practising pranayama that he decided to dedicate his life to researching the therapeutic benefits of different forms of yoga. He and his team work closely with orthodox doctors and carry out clinical

Supported leg raises

This pose provides a gentle stretch and is ideal for those suffering from stiffness. Lie on your back and stretch your legs up against the wall. Stretch your arms above your head and keep your spine stretched. Hold for as long as you are comfortable.

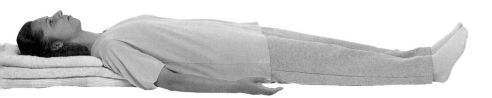

Find out more

Yoga	*46–47*
Relaxation	*58–59*
Choosing a practitioner 106–107	

research in major British teaching hospitals. The idea is to analyse this ancient discipline by modern clinical research methods, to discover exactly how and why it works, and how it can best be adapted to give maximum relief for intractable conditions. Based at the Royal Homeopathic Hospital in London, the Yoga Therapy Centre offers a specialized eight-week course designed for sufferers of all forms of arthritis.

Yoga therapy is very different from ordinary yoga, as the therapy has been adapted and modified for arthritis sufferers. A distinction is made between osteoarthritis, which afflicts mainly older people and is caused by wear and tear on the joints, and rheumatoid arthritis, which affects the whole body and can result in eye and heart problems as well as stiff, painful, inflamed joints.

The benefits of yoga

If you have arthritis, you tend not to work the joints and, as a result, they become ever stiffer and more painful. Although drug treatment can ease the pain, it does not usually restore mobility. One of the main benefits of yoga for arthritis is that sufferers learn to work their joints again. The reason that joints can start to work is that correct movement is accompanied by special yogic breathing and relaxation. Because it is so specialized, yoga therapy – both

Corpse pose

This pose aids complete relaxation of mind and body. Lie on your back with your legs and arms straight, but not tense. Rest your head on a folded towel or blanket. Take a few deep gentle breaths, then let your breathing become slow and even. Stay in this position for at least 15 minutes.

breathing and exercises – must be taught by people who have undergone specific training courses. It would suit those who like getting out, who enjoy being part of a class, and who would welcome the challenge of learning something new.

Once the joints start working again, sufferers can often increase their range of movement. Everybody can manage something, even if it is only working the feet and hands very slightly.

Supported corpse pose

This is a particularly restful pose for the back. Lie on your back with your hand resting on a folded towel or blanket. Support your legs, bent at the knee, on a level chair or stool. Breathe evenly, and rest in this position for several minutes. (If you find you are distracted, close your eyes for concentration.)

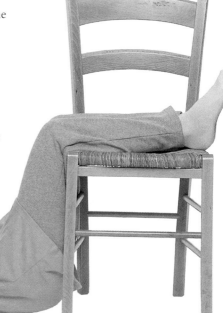

Yoga

A therapy for everyone

People tend to think they shouldn't do yoga if they have arthritis, but research has shown that even the most severely crippled sufferer can do some form of yoga with no adverse effects.

The exercises are very gentle, unlike the strong yogic movements aimed at healthy bodies, and can be adapted for use by those in wheelchairs.

The beneficial effect of yoga therapy is not confined to the joints. Yoga enables circulation to improve and, although it cannot reverse arthritis once the condition has set in, it can help to prevent further accumulation of waste matter in the joints. Yoga also keeps the muscles utilized, and helps drainage of toxins from the lymphatic system.

Patients start feeling better after just one session and, by contrast with orthodox medicine, the only side-effects are good ones. The more you practise yoga, the more beneficial the therapy proves to be. Ideally, arthritis sufferers should practise gentle yoga daily, never going beyond the limits of what they have been taught in classes.

Yoga therapy has also been found to have a beneficial effect on the depression and anxiety that can so often accompany arthritis. All chronic pain causes depression, and, although you can get anti-depressants, this just means putting more drugs with potential side-effects into your body. An important aspect of yoga is the body–mind approach. It works as a kind of cognitive therapy.

An ongoing practice

There is no need to tell your doctor if you are attending yoga therapy, although you should let your physician know about any alternative treatments. Patients are strongly advised to continue with any medication they may be on. Yoga will not interfere with any anti-arthritis medication you may be taking.

After finishing a course, patients must continue to practise at home, perhaps

CASE HISTORY

In 1974, Suzanne was severely injured in a road accident. As she recovered, she started to develop arthritis. Doctors warned her that she would probably never regain full use of her limbs. She became interested in yoga after watching it on television, and then decided to give it a try.

"I started attending regular yoga classes, and soon felt the life energy flood through me. The main thing is that I regained confidence in my body and I was able to learn conscious relaxation.

"Now I practise yoga regularly. Every time I feel any stiffness or immobility in my joints, I breathe into the affected areas. My own feeling is that with arthritis, the most important aspect of the therapy is relaxation. Yoga keeps the joints mobile and free-moving, and it works the whole body.

"I was in my twenties when the accident happened and am convinced that if it hadn't been for regular yoga practice, I would be completely crippled by now, and most likely I would be permanently confined in a wheelchair."

returning every now and again for a refresher course. You can't really learn yoga therapy in a few weeks, you have to build it into your life. The amount of movement you will get back into your joints depends on how severe the arthritis was to begin with.

There is no guaranteed method of preventing arthritis, but there is now some research to show that those who have practised yoga for many years are less likely to suffer from the condition, at least in its severest, most debilitating form.

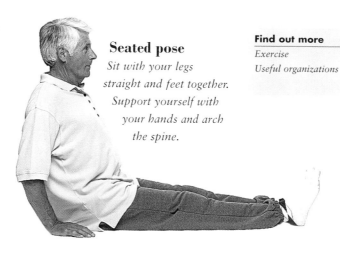

Seated pose

Sit with your legs straight and feet together. Support yourself with your hands and arch the spine.

Find out more

Exercise	148–151
Useful organizations	155

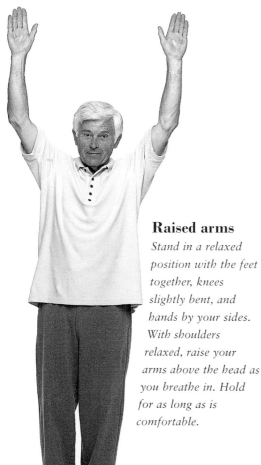

Raised arms

Stand in a relaxed position with the feet together, knees slightly bent, and hands by your sides. With shoulders relaxed, raise your arms above the head as you breathe in. Hold for as long as is comfortable.

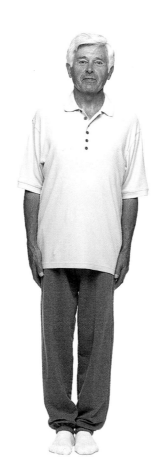

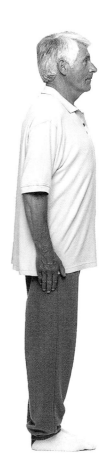

Basic standing posture

Keep a relaxed stance and breathe into the abdomen. Let the shoulders relax. Bring the neck back and the hips forward to maintain a straight spine. Your weight should be centred on the balls of the feet.

T'ai chi ch'uan

T'ai chi ch'uan – usually shortened to t'ai chi – is one of a group of non-combative, gentle martial arts that developed in China and Japan. It is a system of physical and mental training that is used for achieving understanding of the self, expressed through physical movement and self-defence. T'ai chi is used as part of a quest for improved health, both spiritual and physical.

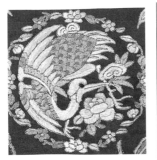

In Taoist philosophy, the crane represents universal consciousness.

The Chinese system of t'ai chi is said to date back many centuries when a Taoist monk, Chang San Feng, invented the movements seen today after dreaming about a strange part-fight, part-dance between a snake and a bird. The traditional postures express the blending of the eternal and the present, heaven and earth.

When Mao Zedong came to power in China in 1949, he proposed t'ai chi ch'uan as a universal health practice to be carried out every morning. The traditional postures were simplified to 24 movements to make it easier for the population to adopt.

Arthritis and t'ai chi

Advocates of t'ai chi point out that it increases oxygen flow to the blood and

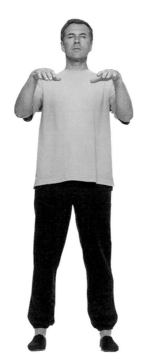

2 *Keeping your knees unlocked and abdomen relaxed, raise your arms slowly to chest height, turning your palms downward. Allow your fingers to open slightly.*

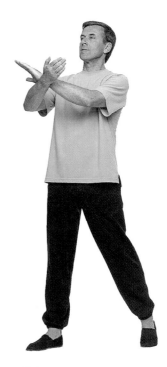

3 *Bring your arms across your chest. Push with your right leg to shift your body weight onto your left foot. As you do so, and your weight comes forward, allow your arms to straighten from the elbow.*

1 *Stand with your feet shoulder width apart and facing forward. Relax your arms and shoulders.*

opens out the joints of the body, especially the knees, alleviating inflammatory diseases such as arthritis. Relief from pain, always an important concern for the arthritis sufferer, is just one of the benefits that t'ai chi offers.

The most appealing factors for arthritis sufferers lie in the ability of t'ai chi to harmonize body and mind, to restore balance to the systems of the body, to boost the immune system, to improve the circulation, to boost energy flow and to begin the process of eliminating toxins from the muscles and joints of the body. All this can be done in a peaceful, gentle fashion without imposing any further strain on the beleaguered body.

Learn from a professional

You will benefit most from t'ai chi by learning the postures from a recognized teacher and you can choose to learn as many or as few postures as you personally feel able to cope with. Practising 24 postures daily will benefit your overall health.

Each of the postures, including the repetitions, takes some 20 minutes to perform. You may be encouraged to learn the short form of some of the postures as each one takes only about five to ten minutes to perform. Once you have learned the required postures, you will be able to practise t'ai chi alone at home, in your garden or in a public space.

Find out more

Choosing a practitioner 106–107
Exercise   148–151

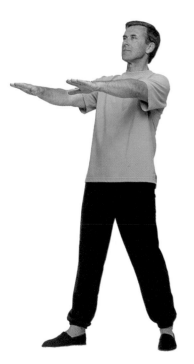 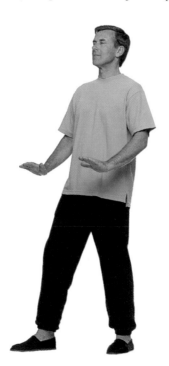 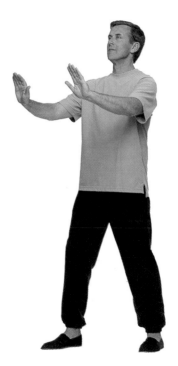

4 *Keeping your elbows slightly bent and facing downward, move your hands outward and away from each other until your arms are in line with your shoulders and your fingers are facing forward.*

5 *Slowly transfer your weight back to your right foot, bending your knee. Keep your back straight. Bring your hands back toward your waist so that the space between them gradually widens. Lift the toes of your left foot.*

6 *Push with your right foot so that your weight is transferred to your left foot and your lower left leg is almost vertical. Move your hands forward and up until they are in line with your shoulders.*

Aromatherapy

It has been known for centuries that certain aromatic oils distilled from plants possess many dramatic healing properties. Most of us are now familiar with aromatherapy as a beauty and relaxation treatment. Aromatherapy products are readily available in the form of massage or bath oils.

Essential oils should be extracted from the leaves, petals, seeds, roots or bark of plants through a process of cold pressing, or steam distillation. No other chemicals or additives should be used in the extraction process.

The ancient Egyptians, with their love of sensuality and rich perfumes, are usually regarded as the founders of aromatherapy. They used aromatic oils for massage, healing and embalming, and Egyptian mummies owe their extraordinary preservation to the powers of plant essences. In fact, archaeologists have identified cedarwood and myrrh aromas lingering in the bandages of mummies that are 3,000 years old.

The ancient art was revived in France in the 1920s when a chemist, René Gattefossé, rediscovered the powerful antiseptic properties of certain aromatic plants. While working in his laboratory, his hand was severely burned following an explosion, and he plunged it into a nearby dish of lavender essence. Gattefossé was astonished at how quickly the wound healed. As a result, he decided to undertake serious research into the medicinal properties of essential oils. His findings were published in 1928 in a book called *Aromatherapie* – a term coined by Gattefossé.

Aromatherapy today

The founder of modern clinical aromatherapy was Jean Valnet, an orthodox-trained French doctor and army surgeon who used essential oils to treat the burns and wounds of soldiers during the Second World War. Dr Valnet discovered that certain oils had the power to alleviate psychiatric conditions, such as shell-shock, that were brought on by the trauma of modern warfare.

Dr Valnet was one of the first doctors to use essential oils internally and, in France to this day, aromatherapy is used widely by conventional doctors and is considered to be part of mainstream medicine.

The power of certain essential oils to relieve arthritis and rheumatic pains was discovered by accident, as a welcome but unexpected side-effect of treatment with plant essences.

The Austrian biochemist Marguerite Maury, who practised mainly in France, was one of the first therapists to use aromatherapy as a holistic mind and

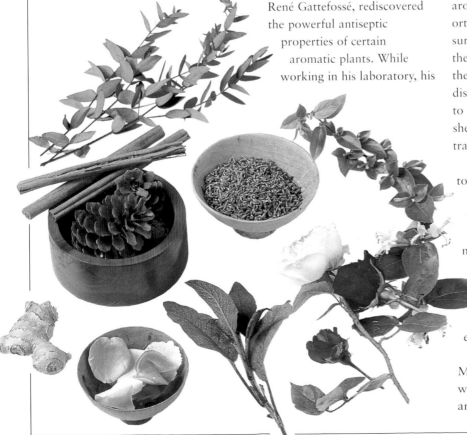

body treatment. Her work was inspired by Gattefossé, but she added a special massage technique which consisted of applying essential oils along the nerve centres of the spine.

Although Mme Maury was treating mainly wealthy clients seeking merely rejuvenation, a number started reporting dramatic improvements in their rheumatic and arthritic pains. These effects lasted weeks or even months after the treatments had finished. One of Marguerite Maury's outstanding pupils was Daniele Ryman, who runs a pioneering aromatherapy clinic in London, and has continued Maury's clinical work.

What are essential oils?

Essential oils are volatile, aromatic liquid components of strong-smelling plants. These liquids are found in different areas, depending on the plant. They may be found in petals (as with roses), leaves (eucalyptus, bay), wood (sandalwood) or bark, fruit (lemon, orange), seeds (caraway, black pepper), roots (sassafras), rhizomes (ginger) or resin (pine). Sometimes, aromatics are found in more than one plant component. Lavender, for example, produces aromatic oils in both its flowers and its leaves. The orange tree is particularly useful in this respect as it yields aromatic essences from the blossom, leaves and fruit.

Plants produce essential oils not primarily to perfume and enhance the lives of humans, but for their own survival. Some oils may influence growth and production, some may attract insects or repel predators, and others are for the purpose of protection from disease.

Genuine aromatherapy oils are usually expensive, and the main reason for this is that you need many petals, roots or leaves to produce even a tiny amount of essential oil. The oils are highly concentrated (you should *never* use neat aromatherapy oil on the skin) and a little lasts for a long time.

Modern laboratory analysis has revealed that essential oils have a complex chemistry. They consist of hundreds of different components, many of which have not yet been fully analysed.

Healing with oils

So how can these aromatic oils relieve and soothe arthritis? Over the centuries, it has been discovered that essential oils possess a number of therapeutic properties. As they are primarily present in the plant for survival purposes, they are all antiseptic. At the same time, some possess anti-viral or anti-inflammatory properties. The oils promote natural healing in the body by stimulating and reinforcing the body's own healing mechanisms. They act directly on the central nervous system, and different oils have different qualities.

Some essences encourage relaxation; others stimulation. Certain oils have the ability to normalize the body's symptoms. Garlic, for example, usually taken in the form of pills rather than as an adjunct to massage, can both raise low blood pressure and reduce high blood pressure.

Essential oils have the ability to ease arthritis on a number of levels. In the first instance, the correct oils can calm inflammation and lessen pain. They reduce muscle tension, which may add to arthritic pain. Secondly, there is – as with so many complementary treatments – a dramatic mind–body effect, as many oils have the power to help alleviate anxiety, depression and anger.

Aromatherapy

An aromatherapy massage promotes relaxation, which can be difficult to achieve when you are trying to cope with the pain, stiffness and immobility of a severe arthritic condition. Massage with essential oils also makes you feel cosseted, cared for and soothed – all positive states of mind which can powerfully aid the physical healing process.

As with other complementary treatments, aromatherapy cannot cure arthritis, but it may relieve or improve the condition. As the effects can be strong, your aromatherapist should ideally be someone who has been trained to treat arthritis sufferers. An aromatherapy massage should be viewed as a medical – rather than a beauty – treatment.

The stress factor

Aromatherapists believe that essential oils affect our health primarily at the level of the mind and the emotions. The many chemicals in the oils directly influence our brains to promote positive thinking and optimism. Relief of stress sets the healing process in motion and alleviates any physical problems that may have resulted from stress and tension being held for a long time in the emotions.

Patricia Davis, another pioneer of aromatherapy as a medical treatment, developed severe arthritis at the early age of 26. She was prescribed drugs that were later found to be dangerous, and her condition gradually worsened. The combination of a healthy balanced diet and aromatherapy relieved her arthritis.

When Davies trained as an aromatherapist in the 1960s, the treatment was derided by orthodox doctors. Times have changed, and aromatherapy is now widely accepted.

If you are interested in using essential oils to treat arthritis, it is advisable to book an initial consultation with a qualified aromatherapist who can recommend a holistic regime appropriate for your particular condition, lifestyle and inclinations. Their professional organization can put you in touch with suitably qualified aromatherapists.

Aromatherapy oils must always be diluted in a carrier oil before being applied to the skin (two to three drops essential oil to 10–20 ml/2–3 tsp carrier is usually sufficient, but check with a qualified aromatherapist if you are unsure). These formulations can then be applied on a compress.

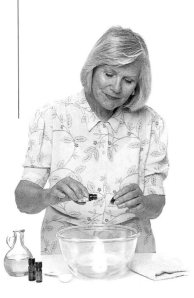
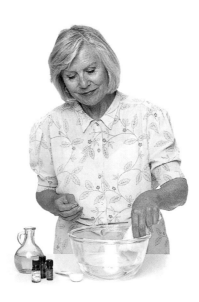
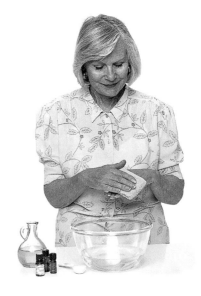

OILS FOR ARTHRITIS

The following aromatherapy oils and essences have been found helpful to assuage the pain and immobility of arthritis.

Black pepper	Coriander	Lavender	Sweet marjoram
Cajuput	Cypress	Lemon	
Chamomile	Frankincense	Sage	
Clove	Juniper	Sweet thyme	

Note: Aromatherapy oils for medicinal purposes come in very small dark brown or blue bottles with rubber stopper tops. The oils must always be mixed with a suitable carrier oil, such as olive, sunflower or soya, before use and never used directly on the skin. As the oils are extremely volatile, the stopper must always be firmly replaced. Aromatherapy treatments which are ready mixed and can be used directly on the skin are sold in large bottles and are labelled "massage oil".

Find out more

Naturopathy	64–65
Massage	68–73
Daily diets	142–147

Treatments for arthritis

These self-help aromatherapy treatments are suitable for safe, effective home use by arthritis sufferers. They have been devised by Daniele Ryman:

1. Dip a small towel in a basin containing very hot water, mixed with 15 ml (1 tbsp) of cider vinegar, two drops each of pine and cypress oils, and one drop of lavender oil.

Apply this compress morning and night to the affected areas. Follow with an application of olive or nut oil and keep the areas warm.

2. Using a mild, unfragranced body shampoo as a base, make up an emulsion containing one drop each of pine, juniper and cypress oils. Run hot water into the bath, then add the emulsion.

Lie in the bath for as long as possible. Afterward, wrap yourself in a warm towelling dressing gown and rest on your bed for 10 minutes.

Pimento massage oil

This oil is very warming, and can thus help to relieve the pain of arthritis.
You will need:
10 ml (2 tsp) soya oil
2 drops wheatgerm oil
3 drops pimento oil
Mix all ingredients together and apply to affected areas. Massage in well, then cover with a hot compress.

NOTE: Although aromatherapy treatments can help to soothe the pain and inflammation of arthritis, relief is not guaranteed. As with all arthritis treatments, these will help some people more than others. They work best in conjunction with an anti-arthritis diet and a generally holistic, healthy regime.

Warming oils may make the skin somewhat tender after treatment. Rub in neat soya oil to soothe the skin.

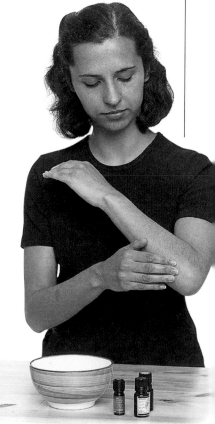

CHAPTER TWO

Meditation

Meditation is the ultimate mind-over-matter therapy. It enables the arthritis sufferer to achieve a deeper level of consciousness and, in doing so, to bring about relief from pain and the everyday problems with which arthritis is associated.

The practice of stilling the mind by conscious effort has been practised in Asia and the Far East for thousands of years. Meditation has become a popular means of coping with the stresses, strains and anxieties of modern life.

Since the 1960s, meditation has been subjected to much scientific investigation to try and discover exactly how it benefits people. Research with EEG machines and other modern equipment has shown conclusively that regular meditation can bring about a profound improvement in the health of both mind and body.

Benefits of meditation

Meditation can achieve increased energy levels, improved concentration, better physical health and relief from pain. It has also been shown that meditation can normalize hormonal activity, increase blood circulation, stimulate the immune system and release muscular tension.

The relaxation response

It is now known that stress of all kinds, including trying to cope with the physical problems of chronic pain, stiffness and immobility, has a severe effect on a wide variety of body functions. When someone is stressed, for whatever reason, the body's arousal systems all go into permanent "red alert" and this results in large amounts of excess adrenaline – the stress hormone – flooding into every cell of the body. This causes a permanent sensation of anxiety and unease which in time you may not be conscious of. When this happens, the ability to relax is impaired, even during periods of sleep.

You do not have to have an image as a focus in order to meditate successfully, but initially many people find that a tranquil image helps to keep stray thoughts at bay.

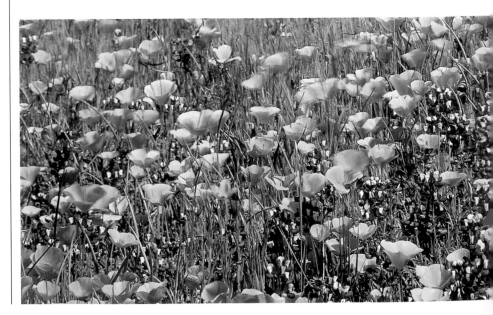

Meditation has the power to reduce stress levels gradually and safely, so that the body's self-healing mechanisms can once more come into operation.

Meditation allows the brain waves to slow down from beta – the normal waking state – to alpha, which is the wave in which healing, creativity and positive thinking take place. In the alpha state, the mind slows down, becomes receptive, and senses rather than thinks.

A commitment to relax

There are no harmful side-effects from meditation, and it can be practised any time, anywhere. However, meditation is an art that has to be learned, and practised daily in order to achieve proficiency. For most people, the art of being relaxed and alert at the same time does not come naturally. It takes persistent effort to learn the techniques.

Nowadays, there are many schools of meditation, and many different ways to meditate. Some people find it easier to do this in a class setting, with somebody guiding the meditation. Others prefer to be alone, and meditation can be learned quite easily at home. It is a good idea to buy a tape to start with, which will guide you through a meditation and stop you becoming bored (or sleepy) until you have mastered the art of relaxed concentration.

You may find that your mind wanders off into thinking about trivial things, such as what's for dinner and compiling a shopping list. One way of keeping the mind still is to focus on something – it could be the flame of a candle or a spiritual picture – and pull yourself back to this every time the mind strays. You do not need to keep your eyes shut.

Meditation has been found to be very effective for pain relief, and is increasingly being used in hospitals, pain clinics and hospices for this purpose. It requires some investment of time with its daily practice, but the dividends, you will probably find, are invaluable. The meditative effect from each session lasts only a few hours, which is why two dedicated sessions every day are recommended.

Find out more

Relaxation	*58–59*
Self-hypnosis	*60–61*
Biofeedback	*99*

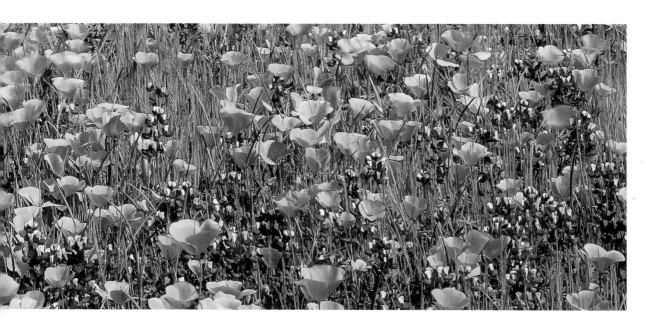

Visualization

Visualization techniques for the relief of serious illness and pain were first developed in the 1960s, when American cancer specialists Carl and Stephanie Simonton discovered that if patients could imagine cancer cells shrinking and fading away, those cells often responded by doing exactly that.

Using your imagination as an adjunct to healing can bring about positive results. Visualization is the ability to imagine yourself well, or successful, and in an optimal state of health. By inducing such a state of mind, there can be profound beneficial effects on the body.

Visualization has become an integral part of complementary cancer care, and it is a therapy that is taught in many cancer hospitals. These techniques can easily be adapted to other serious and chronic illnesses, including arthritis.

With arthritis, visualization would involve seeing twisted, painful joints functioning smoothly and strongly again, and imagining a life without crippling pain and disability.

The results vary depending very much on the personality of the patient. The technique works best for people with good imaginations or for those who are able to allow their minds to express themselves freely. Perhaps for this reason children and young people tend to have more success than older adults, although anyone can achieve good results if they allow their minds such freedom.

Choose a comfortable position – and somewhere you won't be disturbed. Relax, breathe easily, and let your mind roam freely.

Getting prepared

In order to practise creative visualization, you need to sit or lie in the most comfortable position for you. Then be still and let your mind settle. Now you can start to give your imagination free rein, and try to think of all the ways in which you would like your life to improve. Indulge in as many fantasies as you like.

Try to imagine you are in a place where you feel happy and content. For example, some people like to see themselves by the sea, with the sun warming them. Gradually become part of the scene. See yourself as fit and well, totally pain-free and with a positive and happy outlook on life.

After a while, pinpoint the one particular area of your life in which you would especially welcome change. Try to see in your mind an image of how you would like yourself to be, and, as you do so, begin to believe that this will happen.

The process could take as little as 30 seconds, but it usually requires a few minutes. When you have focused on your greatest needs, start to think about how – and whether – these are being met.

Affirmations

The next step is to make some affirmations. These can be written or spoken, but they must always be expressed in the present tense, rather than the future.

One affirmation could be: "I am well and my joints are supple and mobile." Or, you could put it a different way and say: "I am now attracting wellness and mobility into my life."

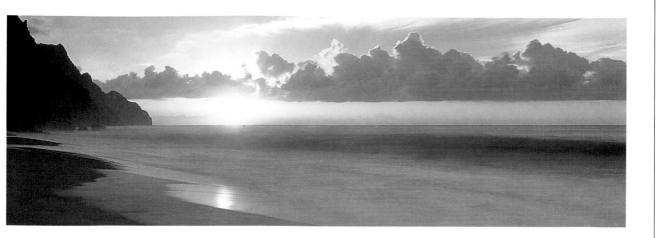

Visualization, in common with other conscious mental techniques, works by a very specific mechanism. First decide what you want to create, and then give yourself a mental picture of the result. The more often you repeat the process, the stronger will be your focus and concentration on the goal, and the better your chances of bringing about the desired result. Affirmations rely on the same technique, reinforcement. Eventually, you learn by simple repetition exactly what you are striving for and, in turn, what you will do to achieve that.

Practical exercises

Try the following visualizations for improved physical health:

1. Relax as much as possible.
   Now try to project your consciousness into your foot.
   Explore how much of your foot you can sense with your mind.
   Now slowly start to do the same with your legs.
   Feel them in your mind.
   Gradually work your way up your body and as you do this, try to see images of the inside of your body.
   Visualize everything in turn as being well and strong.

2. This "white light" visualization works well for serious illness.
   First, sit down with your back as straight as possible.
   Now try to visualize a pool of white light at the base of your spine.
   Take a deep breath and hold for a couple of seconds.
   As you breathe out, visualize this white light shooting up your spine and out of the top of your head. As it does this, the healing light cascades over your whole body.
   Repeat the exercise.
   Every time you exhale, feel this intense pure light shooting up your spine and pouring down your body like divine rain, healing everywhere it touches.

3. Arthritis sufferers need to develop the habit of visualizing the diseased areas as being strong and healthy with all the joints functioning smoothly. Visualize yourself walking without pain, running even, and imagine all the things that you would like to do with your strong, healthy body.

It is the amount of energy or life force behind the image together with the reinforcement technique that brings about the desired improvement.

As a prelude to any visualization exercise, you may like to picture yourself in a pleasant, tranquil setting. This can be an effective way to calm the mind.

Relaxation

R elaxation therapy does not yield its full benefit in a day or even a week. However, once you have practised relaxation techniques systematically for several weeks, you may well gain a considerable degree of pain relief and improved mobility.

Holding stress and tension in the body for a long time sets up many adverse physical reactions in the system. You will feel considerably drained of energy, for instance, muscle tension is increased, your blood pressure is likely to be raised and the circulation is hampered.

Relaxation techniques that work to calm the nervous system and release muscle tension are an excellent way of coping with the pain of arthritis without taking more painkillers. The ability to relax will also help all the other body systems to normalize.

Learn to breathe

Tensing up against constant pain promotes poor posture and disturbs digestion, but above all it can lead to hyperventilation, a type of shallow breathing rather like panting that eventually disturbs the chemical composition of every cell in the body, and puts the system into perpetual panic mode.

It is impossible to relax unless you are breathing deeply and slowly. For many people who have become used to being in constant pain, this takes a good deal of practice to achieve.

Breathing exercise

Try this easy method of building relaxed breathing into your life.

First of all make yourself as comfortable as possible, and try to ensure that your weight is evenly distributed on both sides of your body. The more symmetry you can attain, the easier

A TECHNIQUE WITH MUSIC

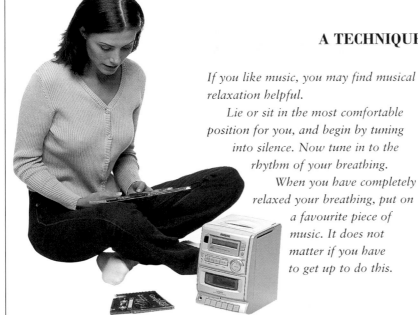

If you like music, you may find musical relaxation helpful.

Lie or sit in the most comfortable position for you, and begin by tuning into silence. Now tune in to the rhythm of your breathing.

When you have completely relaxed your breathing, put on a favourite piece of music. It does not matter if you have to get up to do this.

As the music starts, begin to breathe into it and allow yourself to absorb the rhythms completely. Continue to breathe deeply and slowly for the duration of the piece of music.

When the music comes to an end, don't come out of your state abruptly or rush to do other things: continue your relaxation for a few minutes, easing yourself back into your normal waking state and normal surroundings slowly and gently.

relaxed breathing will become. Turn off any main lights and make sure that your immediate environment is as quiet and serene as you can make it.

Now close your eyes and pay conscious attention to your breathing. Allow each breath to become longer, slower and deeper. Breathe deeply into the abdomen, pushing your stomach out as you breathe and letting it sink back down again as you breathe out.

With each inhalation, repeat to yourself: "Deep and long and slow" and with each exhalation, repeat "slow and long and deep". You may find your mind wandering, but every time it does, bring it back to your breathing again.

As the lungs continue to breathe deeper, longer and slower, become aware of how the whole of your body begins to breathe deeper, longer and slower as well. As you inhale, imagine pure energy flooding in. As you exhale, imagine the pain flooding out.

To end the relaxation, move your body gently, open your eyes, sit up and, lastly, stand up very carefully.

Try to practise this relaxed breathing for five minutes at first, gradually building up the time as you get used to it.

Find out more

Meditation	*54–55*
Biofeedback	*99*

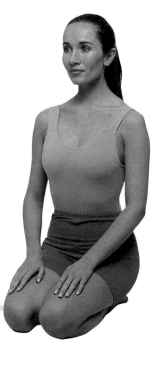

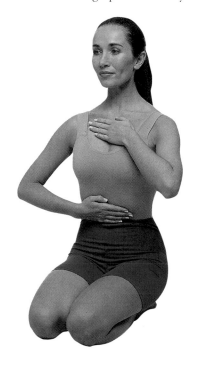

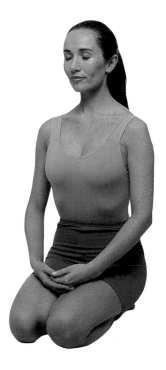

1 *Sit in a position that is comfortable. Some people are happy sitting cross-legged; others prefer sitting back on their heels. Alternatively you can sit in a chair, preferably one with an upright back, or lie on a mat on the floor.*

2 *Place your right hand on your abdomen just below your ribcage, and your left hand in the centre of your upper chest. When you are breathing abdominally, your lower hand should move in and out and your upper hand should be motionless.*

3 *Rest your hands in your lap with thumbs lightly touching. Count to 10 as you breathe in through your noses, hold the breath for a few seconds and slowly exhale. Repeat this 10 times. If any distractions slip into your mind, let them float in and float out again.*

Self-hypnosis

Self-hypnosis may sound exotic, but it is, at least in its medical sense, more a form of very deep relaxation than the ability to put yourself into a trance. The point about this form of healing is that when you have reached a deeply relaxed state, you can give yourself instructions which the mind and body will obey.

Focusing on a regularly repeated pattern such as a flight of stairs or a tree-lined avenue may help your efforts at self-hypnosis: each stair brings you one step closer to a state of total relaxation.

Over the past few years, self-hypnosis techniques have been used with great success to reduce pain, including the pain of arthritis. In particular, self-hypnosis has been shown in a number of clinical trials to be very effective for people who suffer chronic pain which is not easily alleviated by drugs or surgery, and which is always likely to return. So as an arthritis sufferer, self-hypnosis might work for you.

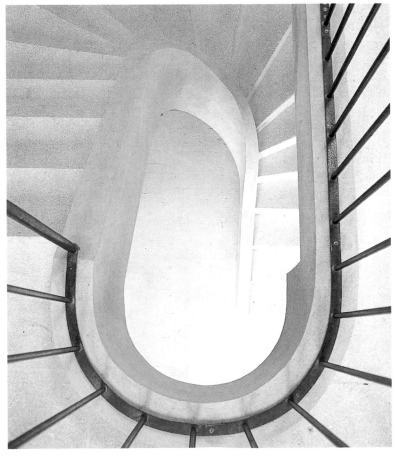

Are you a good subject?

Most experts now define the hypnotized state as a distinct level of consciousness somewhere between waking and deep sleep, in which the subject experiences an altered state of reality. When in a state of hypnosis, your conscious mind is submerged beneath the threshold of pain, and you are able to access your inner calm.

Self-hypnosis is not as difficult or strange as you may imagine, and many people find they are able to do it. Answer the following questions to discover if you might benefit from this technique:
• Do you tend to cry at sad films?
• Are you liable to miss your stop on the bus or train because you are completely engrossed in a book?
• Can you fall asleep easily and quickly?
• Can you imagine yourself being in love?
• Do you daydream easily?

If you are able to answer "yes" to these questions, you are potentially a good subject for self-hypnosis.

A simple exercise

To practise self-hypnosis for pain control, try this deep relaxation exercise. First choose a time and place where you will not be disturbed, and you have no pressing concerns. Unplug your telephone or put on your answering machine.

Now close your eyes and relax your breathing. As you relax, breathe more and more deeply.

Relax all your muscles except those used for breathing. Imagine that you can feel every molecule of air flowing in and out of your body. Keep breathing ever more deeply. Consciously try to make every breath exactly the same length, so that you become more and more deeply relaxed with each breath out. Imagine a wave of perfect relaxation flowing slowly throughout your whole body.

Once you are perfectly relaxed, try to identify exactly where your pain is and what triggers it off. When you have done this, make some strong pain-control affirmations to your unconscious. You may want to use your own affirmations, but here are some suggestions you could try: "My neck muscles are bathed and soothed by perfect warmth" or "My legs are warm and relaxed whenever I go for a walk." An affirmation such as "My joints are becoming more supple and less stiff all the time" may work for you.

You might like to try a variation on this exercise. Follow the same steps to achieve a state of deep relaxation. Then place a hand over the area where you have pain. Imagine that your hand is relaxed, heavy and numb. Then visualize that these sensations are replacing the feelings of pain.

Monitor your progress

In order for self-hypnosis to be effective, you need to make the effort to measure your pain levels. Try to analyse your pain – is it the worst you can remember? half as bad? is it bearable? – and devise a "ranking" system. Don't expect magical results at once. This is not stage hypnosis. Professional hypnotherapists explain that hypnosis works to control pain slowly, bit by bit. This is why you need to measure your pain and monitor each small improvement, and to keep practising.

Ideally, you should practise self-hypnosis every day, at the same time, and rate your comfort level after every session, so that you can observe your degree of progress for yourself.

Find out more

Meditation	*54–55*
Relaxation	*58–59*
Managing the pain	*138–141*

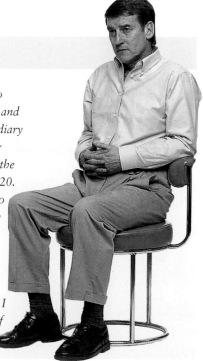

CASE HISTORY

James was advised by his doctor that anti-inflammatory drugs to control the pain of his arthritis were not suitable for him because of his history of stomach ulcers. But, as the pain was so severe, he had to do something to relieve it, and James found that self-hypnosis provided the answer.

"I was sceptical at first, but I was in such pain that I was desperate to do anything that might help. I came across a book on self-hypnosis, and realized I had nothing to lose by trying it.

"It took dedication and practice, but to my amazement after about a month of daily practice it started to work – I found I was able to relax and begin to control the pain. I kept a diary of my level of pain before and after each 20-minute session, and noted the improvements on a scale of one to 20.

"This gave me the motivation to continue, and I find that I can now actually eliminate the pain by this means. Of course, self-hypnosis is not a cure, and the pain keeps returning. But I'm sure it's at least as effective as drugs would be, and I feel that I have a certain measure of control over the pain."

Professional help

One of the advantages of consulting a complementary practitioner rather than relying on self-help remedies is that your progress will be objectively monitored, and your regular weekly or monthly visit will give a structure and a discipline to your treatment.

There are many excellent reasons to consult a complementary therapist, but perhaps most important is that you will have an opportunity to discuss your arthritis with somebody friendly who is interested in helping you. This is especially useful if, for example, you find it difficult to maintain your motivation with self-help treatments such as meditation or visualization.

Complementary practitioners provide essential support and guidance. Many therapists are happy to work in conjunction with your orthodox treatment, to provide back-up, comfort and additional holistic care. One major benefit of seeing a therapist is that most practitioners prefer to take their time with their patients: you are unlikely to feel as if you are on a conveyor belt. This can in itself be helpful and healing when you are trying to cope with a chronic illness.

As there are so many therapies on offer, you can choose the one, or the combination, that best suits your mobility, pain level, outlook and pocket. Bear in mind that some of these therapies can become expensive over time. You will probably have to attend a clinic or consulting room, although in some cases the therapist may come to your home. Clinics vary enormously. The formal look of a clinic is not necessarily a guide to the quality of advice and treatment you can expect, and the therapist may or may not be registered (see pp.42–43).

Practitioner-administered therapies fall into two distinct categories: the hands-on approach, and those performed through a medium of drugs, pills or potions, or advice on diet and exercise. Only you can decide whether you are happy to be touched as part of your treatment regime. You must also decide whether you would prefer a one-to-one personal treatment, or whether you would rather attend a class.

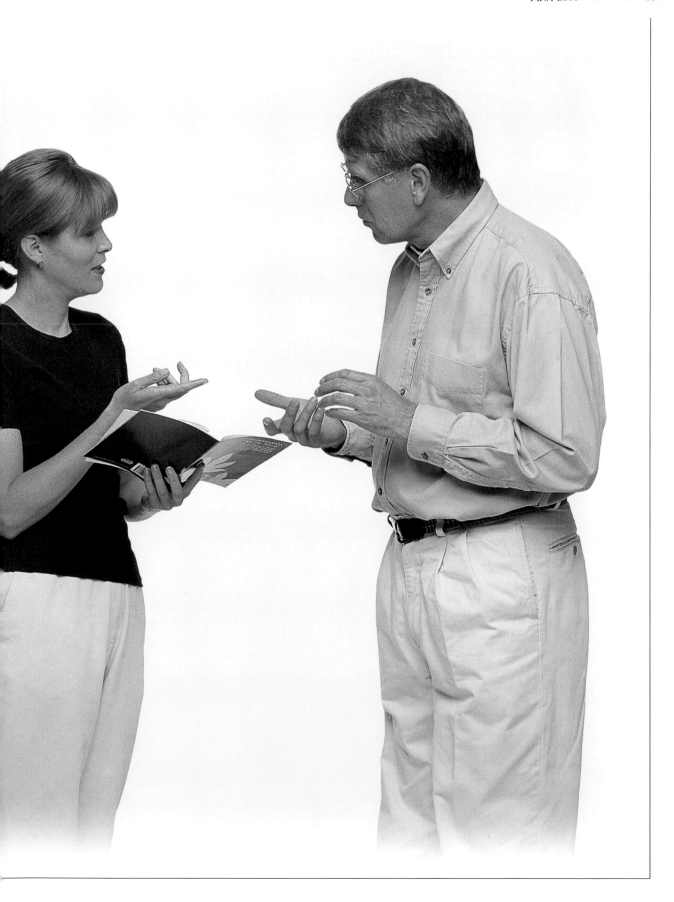

Naturopathy

*N*aturopathy *comprises a common-sense attitude to health based on the body's own healing capabilities. The principal elements of naturopathy are natural resources, including fresh air and sunlight, exercise, rest, good nutrition, hygiene, relaxation and hydrotherapy (water therapy).*

Clean, fresh air, exercise and sunlight are among the factors that can contribute to a general state of wellbeing and good health.

The naturopathic way of life means people taking responsibility for their own health and its very simplicity makes this easily possible. Naturopaths believe that what mainstream doctors regard as symptoms of disease are frequently indications of the body's attempts to reject disease and to throw off the toxic accumulations – the poisoning – that an unhealthy way of life has produced. They further believe that the body has the power to heal itself provided that it is properly treated and maintained.

Naturopaths attempt to remove obstacles to the normal functioning of the body, such as stress, poor posture and bad diet, and apply treatments which will stimulate or promote natural functioning. In essence, therefore, naturopathy is the promotion of health or the practice of preventative medicine rather than the treating of disease.

A broad approach

Today, many naturopathic practitioners, clinics and residential centres use modern medical diagnostic tools such as X-rays, laboratory tests and so on to assist their work, but the basic approach remains the same as it has for centuries, which is to help the body back into equilibrium by harnessing all the cures and treatments found in nature.

Naturopaths have to undergo a lengthy training that includes anatomy, physiology, microbiology, gynaecology, orthopaedics, clinical nutrition, psychology and iridology as diagnostic tools. They will also have to study natural therapies such as homeopathy, herbal medicine, traditional Chinese medicine, hydrotherapy and manipulative techniques such as osteopathy.

This complex training means that naturopaths can offer a range of treatments tailored to your individual requirements.

Naturopathic theory

There are three ruling principles in naturopathy.
1. Naturopathic practitioners work according to the belief that the body is continually trying to restore health and

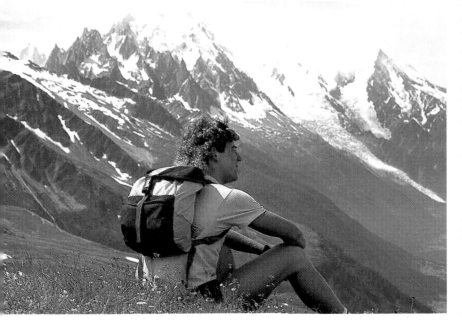

maintain equilibrium, and that all symptoms of pain and distress are attempts to do this. Thus, a naturopath would see the pain and inflammation of arthritis as attempts to return to health. The pain exists to alert you that there is something wrong, and inflammation occurs when the joints are trying to protect themselves against further harm.
2. Naturopaths believe that the underlying cause of all disease is the unwanted accumulation of waste products, and the body's inability to dispose of these naturally and safely. This accumulation is caused by poor lifestyle habits, for example, bad diet, junk food, lack of exercise and lack of fresh air.
3. The third naturopathic principle is that the body actually contains all the wisdom and power it needs to heal itself. It just has to be given the chance.

Your consultation

When you visit a naturopath, you may be prescribed controlled fasting, massage, enemas or colonic irrigation to detoxify the system and help the body to start cleaning itself out. Enzyme therapy, which enables the body to absorb nutrients in food, may be recommended. Many arthritis sufferers are not able to make full use of the nutrients the body takes in, so they may be prescribed freeze-dried plant enzymes in supplement form. The most common of these are bromelain from pineapples and papain from papaya. The naturopath may diagnose your nutritional status by carrying out a blood test or hair mineral analysis.

Many people with arthritis have a history of poor diet, and this will usually have to be amended first. Vitamins A and E are powerful anti-oxidants, and work to destroy the harmful free radicals that accumulate to cause damage around the joints. Vitamin E, in particular, enhances the production of cartilage and helps to reduce inflammation and destruction of joint tissue.

Therapeutics on offer vary from practitioner to practitioner, but they may include using light, water, ultrasound, electricity, heat and cold. There may be exercise techniques such as yoga or breathing techniques; chiropractic, reflexology or massage; biofeedback; and herbal or homeopathic remedies.

Expect a detailed medical and life history to be taken. In some cases, laboratory tests or X-rays may be ordered. However, the most important aspect of a naturopathic consultation is the patient's diet. You may have a previously undetected food allergy that could affect your symptoms, and you will almost certainly be advised to cut down on tea, coffee, colas, alcohol, refined sugars and, possibly, wheat and dairy produce as well.

After the initial consultation, your therapist will discuss the various possibilities for treatment with you, and arrive at the package that seems the most suitable for your individual condition.

Some naturopaths use a technique called hair mineral analysis. A sample of hair is processed in a laboratory to test for any imbalances, which may then be corrected by an appropriate diet.

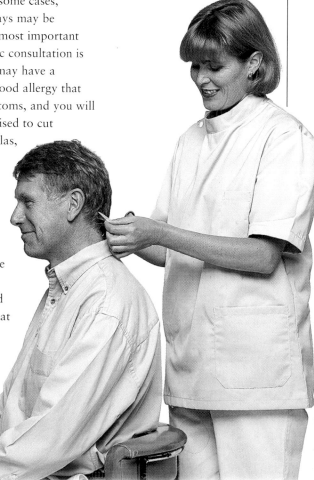

Hydrotherapy

W hen the body is immersed in water, there is less strain on the weight-bearing joints, and this gives a feeling of comfort, relaxation and lightness of being. This takes place in both cold and hot water. Professional hydrotherapy for arthritis, however, is typically carried out in a hot pool.

It has been known since before Roman times that water therapy can bring benefit and relief for arthritis. Hydrotherapy was developed in Austrian Silesia (now part of the Czech Republic) in the early 19th century, by Vincent Preissnitz at his "water university". Toward the end of that century a Bavarian priest, Sebastian Kneipp, classified the therapeutic uses of water and today some centres still offer "Kneipptherapie". Today, it is available at many hospitals and clinics.

Hydrotherapy originally involved the use of spring waters, many of which were rich in minerals, and could be naturally warm or cool. Today, ordinary water is often used, but minerals may still be added in some spas.

How it works
Hydrotherapy, an increasingly popular treatment for arthritis conditions of all kinds, works in two distinct but related ways. Firstly, it gives instant relief of pain and a sense of increased wellbeing and, secondly, being immersed in water allows greater joint mobility while you are actually in the water. For this reason, hydrotherapy is almost always combined with gentle exercise while the joints have this increased mobility. After the exercise session, more hydrotherapy encourages the joints and muscles to relax in a soothing, comforting way.

Relaxing in a hot bath is a form of hydrotherapy in itself, but special hydrotherapy pools are available for use by arthritis sufferers. These are hotter than ordinary swimming pools, and are staffed by physiotherapists or other health-care professionals who are expert in treating this condition.

Specialized care
Hydrotherapy and exercise sessions should be carried out under the supervision of a health-care professional. Otherwise, there is a risk that the joints will be exercised beyond their natural capacity, resulting in more harm than good.

For the treatment to be effective, it is important that the water should be at the correct temperature, as water that is too hot or too cold will not be beneficial and may even restrict mobility. This especially applies if a joint is acutely inflamed. In addition, the skin can be damaged by water that is too hot. For this treatment, you need to book a session or course of sessions at a hydrotherapy pool.

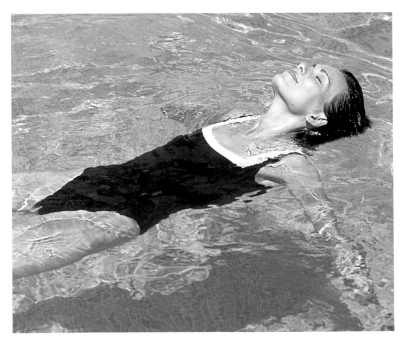

TARGETING RELIEF

Although many arthritis sufferers benefit from whole-body immersion, therapists may choose to work only those areas of the body which are affected, such as the joints of the fingers.

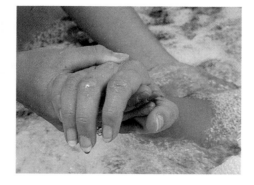

Find out more

Physical therapies   116–121
Managing the pain   138–141

A visit to a spa

Some spas and health farms have pools that are adapted for arthritis sufferers. Treatment in adapted pools or baths may be combined with a hot seaweed or mud wrap afterward to reduce inflammation still further. You might want to consider taking a holiday at one of the residential spas with a proven record for arthritis relief. One of the best known of these is at the Dead Sea, in Israel and Jordan, where specialized clinics staffed by qualified doctors can treat arthritis in its many forms.

The mineral salts and heat in the Dead Sea combine to have a powerful healing effect on inflamed joints. The Dead Sea is the lowest place on the surface of the earth, and the only place where you can sunbathe safely all day without burning. This is because the sun's rays are filtered through the vapours of many salts above the sea's surface.

Many natural hot pools and sulphur pools have specialized arthritis clinics attached to them, and more and more people are discovering that this natural relief can last far longer than the pain relief obtained with pills.

At some spas in the Czech Republic, where scientific research has been carried out on arthritis sufferers, it has been found that hydrotherapy treatment in natural hot pools can give complete pain relief for up to a year. For many arthritis sufferers, that is a welcome prospect.

For relief from severe arthritis, you would probably need to stay at a spa for about three weeks. Although you may derive some relief instantly, you will probably find that the effect does not last long with just one session.

It seems that if you can have hydrotherapy every day, the effect is cumulative. Many spas (although not all) combine hydrotherapy sessions with a healthy diet, perhaps with nutritional supplements, and the opportunity to relax in a beautiful and tranquil setting.

Self-help

You can give yourself treatments at home. Dead Sea minerals, and those from other spas, are now available from chemists for home use. These cannot, by law, claim to treat arthritis, but many sufferers find them extremely effective.

Walking by the sea and swimming in the sea have long been known to bring benefits to health and people with arthritis can benefit from this form of hydrotherapy as well. Swimming helps to retain mobility by maintaining muscle strength and the range of movement around a joint.

Massage

Less popular in the West than so-called Swedish massage, Thai massage relies on different manipulation techniques. One of them, shaking, involves pulling on a limb at the same time as it is moved up and down.

Remedial massage appeals to people who enjoy sensual touch for therapeutic purposes. Therapeutic masseurs usually use oil, and the patient lies on a massage table with his or her clothes removed, covered with soft, warm towels so that the only part of the body exposed is that which is currently being massaged.

Essentially, massage is a sensual healing art to be enjoyed, used to produce a sense of wellbeing. Having massage makes you take time out to relax. Massage also improves the circulation and lowers the heart rate, in addition to bringing about real physical benefits to the joints and loosening and stretching the muscles.

All massage techniques involve kneading and stroking, but there are many different types of massage, ranging from very light, gentle stroking to hard pummelling which may, for some people, approach the threshold of pain.

Schools of massage

There is evidence that schools of massage evolved in many parts of the ancient world, but some are more popular than others in the West.

• Swedish massage uses a routine of basic, firm strokes with kneading and tapping over the whole body.

• Lymphatic drainage massage is newer than Swedish massage and is highly specialized. This form concentrates on stimulating the internal organs by activating the various lymphatic points on the body. The idea is to enable long-held toxins to be flushed from the liver, kidneys and colon.

• Medical massage, which was originally developed during the Second World War specifically for amputees and others suffering from serious wounds, concentrates on relieving severe pain.

The history of massage

Massage was probably used by the early Christians as an element of healing in the so-called laying on of hands, but it was eventually condemned by the church as sinful, as it involved one person touching another. In addition, massage as a healing tool suffered considerably, especially in the West, with the advent of scientific or modern medicine.

The art was revived in the early nineteenth century in Sweden when a Stockholm University student, Henri Peter Ling, started to duplicate gymnastic techniques on the massage table, thereby developing the first form of passive exercise.

Ling devised 47 positions and 800 movements, so that those not athletically gifted could enjoy similar physical benefits to professional athletes. At first, the Swedish medical establishment and the government rejected Ling's system, but he eventually obtained a licence to practise therapeutic massage in 1814.

The practice grew in popularity at spas and health clinics, particularly in sports medicine. Until the 1960s and 1970s, therapeutic massage was restricted to athletes, gymnasts and dancers and the wealthy few who could afford to visit health farms and clinics. Otherwise, massage was available only at "massage parlours" and gained a poor reputation.

A modern therapy

The appeal of massage began to broaden during the late 1960s, when California therapists began to use different forms of massage in their bodywork. Initially, the idea was to help people to break down repressions and long-held inhibitions so that their true unrestrained selves could be released. Gradually, however, it was realized that massage had many therapeutic uses, and so the therapy came to be incorporated back into medicine. Most pain clinics now offer massage.

One of the pioneers of medical massage in the West was British therapist Clare Maxwell-Hudson, who began to promote enthusiastically the benefits of massage in the 1960s. After training as a beauty therapist, she began practising as a masseuse when it still had a somewhat dubious image. For her research into massage techniques, Maxwell-Hudson travelled widely, particularly in the East, and saw for herself how people quite naturally massaged each other, and how closely integrated massage was with traditional healing. She began offering relaxing massage to people (mainly women) in their homes. As her work became better known, Maxwell-Hudson established her own massage school and also began massaging seriously ill patients in hospital. This laid the foundations for the role of massage in pain clinics.

Find out more

Massage	*70–73*
Reflexology	*96–98*

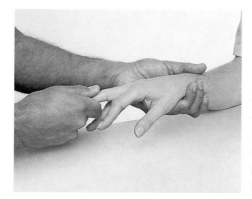

HAND AND FINGER MASSAGE
Massage fingers one at a time, squeezing each between your thumb and finger and sliding along the finger in one stroke.

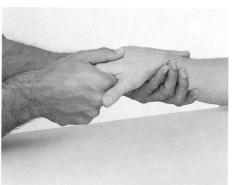

Massage the palm using your thumb, moving it in slow, circular strokes. There are many small, strong muscles in this area, so you may need to apply a firm pressure.

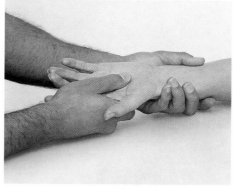

Massage the back of the hand in small, circular movements. Repeat several times over one area before moving on to the next. Use firm pressure, adjusting it to suit the person you are massaging.

Massage

Therapeutic massage

Clare Maxwell-Hudson pioneered therapeutic massage for heart patients at the Charing Cross Hospital in London, at a time when such treatment was considered rather odd. Today, however, massage forms part of conventional treatment for those patients who wish it at hospices, nursing homes, cancer hospitals and AIDS clinics.

"Sometimes, patients are so ill you can only massage their hands," Maxwell-Hudson says. "But even that amount of massage makes them feel better."

Massage has now become so integrated into modern medicine that it constitutes part of British nurses' postgraduate training. In the USA, therapeutic touch is taught at many medical schools, and it has become a branch of medicine in its own right.

Massage can benefit arthritis sufferers in several ways. At the simplest level, there is the fact that gentle stroking over your whole body with aromatic oils makes you feel better. You feel as if somebody cares. At a subtler level, massage also means that somebody accepts your body, and is giving it dedicated attention. Your disabilities, deformities and knotted joints, for a professional masseur, are there to be relieved. Massage can ease the physical aches and pains of arthritis. Therapeutic massage can penetrate knotty joints and muscles and tease them out, helping accumulated toxins to be flushed out from the body.

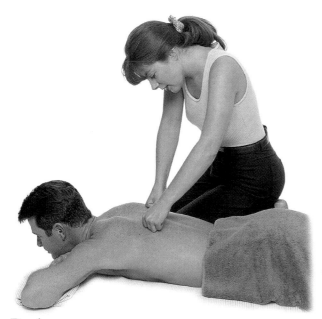

Petrissage

In this technique the hands, fingers or thumbs alternately grasp and loosen specific parts of the body to work on different muscle groups. Petrissage promotes circulation and eases muscle tension.

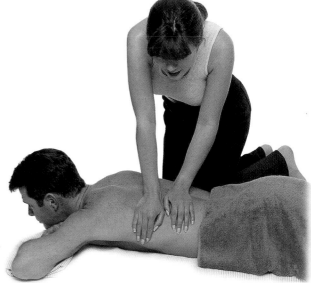

Effleurage

This is a slow, rhythmic, stroking movement applied with the palms of the hands and the fingers. The technique is warming and deeply relaxing and may be used throughout the duration of the massage.

Therapeutic masseurs, especially when working with arthritis or other inflammatory conditions, must fully understand the nature of the condition or they could make the inflammation and wear and tear worse. Professional masseurs undergo rigorous training which includes a detailed knowledge of anatomy and physiology, some psychology, and training on how to deal with patients.

British counsellor and therapist Pat Williams, who teaches listening skills at the Clare Maxwell-Hudson School, says: "In order to be a successful masseur, you not only have to like bodies, whatever their size, shape and condition, but you must also be able to listen very carefully to your patients and clients, and pick up what they need."

The different types of stroke

Four commonly used techniques – petrissage, effleurage, kneading, and tapotement – are described and illustrated below. Other techniques include:
• Touch, that is, putting the hand over a part of the body. This technique is used for very ill people.
• Vibration refers to rapid shaking and pulsating, and this is often done with a machine.
• Brushing indicates a light movement, using just the fingertips. This can tickle, and is used either at the end of a massage, or for people whose medical condition cannot take much pressure.
• Nerve compression refers to firm pressure applied to relieve knots or pain at nerve points.

Find out more

Choosing a practitioner 106–107
Massage   72–73
Reflexology   96–98

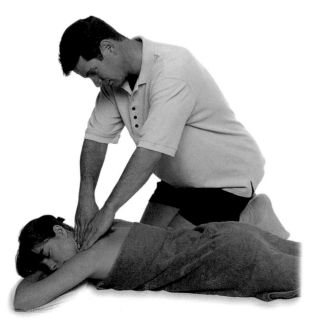

Kneading

In this technique the hands grasp and release often quite large areas of flesh, producing a stimulating and invigorating effect. Kneading helps with the breakdown of fatty tissue and the elimination of toxins from the body.

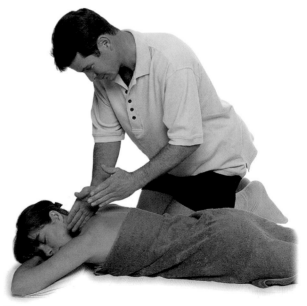

Tapotement

Also called percussion, tapotement is the vigorous striking of broad, fleshy areas of the body using the sides of the hands or loose fists. This stroke helps to improve circulation and is very energizing.

Massage

Massage is increasingly being recognized as a therapy which benefits the mind as well as the body. There are numerous massage products on the market – ranging from aromatherapy oils and tools for self-massage – which make this a very effective and accessible form of therapy.

A visit to a masseur

At your first session, your massage therapist will take a full medical history and ask you questions about your overall health, lifestyle, diet and whether or not you exercise.

You will then be asked to undress and lie down on the couch. The massage room should be warm without being too hot, and most of your body will be covered with warm, dry towels. Only the part of your body currently being massaged will be exposed, and then covered again after.

The session should last for about an hour, by which time you should feel pleasantly relaxed. You will be asked to lie on the massage couch for a few minutes before getting up to leave. It is a good idea to have your massage at a time when you will not have to rush around immediately afterward.

A massage session can either sedate or stimulate, depending on the type of strokes used. Although it is sometimes considered to be a gentle therapy, massage can at times be quite forceful. Men and women who massage athletes and sports competitors use an enormous amount of energy to pummel and coax muscles and tissues into shape.

You should let your masseur know immediately if you feel any undue pain, as this is a warning sign. The strokes used on someone with arthritis tend to be much lighter and gentler than those used on a firm, honed, athletic body.

Most masseurs these days use aromatherapy oils, although some prefer baby oil or even talcum powder. Male masseurs are usually able to apply deeper pressure than women, and some people prefer the large hands of a male masseur. In some clinics, you can get synchronized massage, where two people massage you at the same time for extra effect.

A weekly massage is recommended for the maximum therapeutic effect.

Finding a therapist

As with any medical therapist, it is important that you find a masseur who is properly qualified, with experience and knowledge relevant to your condition. The intimate nature of massage as a therapy means your masseur should be someone with whom you feel comfortable and who inspires your trust.

You can ask your local hospital pain clinic for their list of practitioners or try and obtain a personal recommendation from a friend. Alternatively, your family doctor may know of a medical masseur in your area. Be sure to set your mind at ease and check out your therapist with their governing body (see addresses at the end of the book).

A word of caution

Obviously, massage is a very intimate treatment, usually carried out with just you and the masseur in the room; in addition you are probably naked, although covered up with towels. This can make you feel very vulnerable, especially if it is your first time, and it is the masseur's job to put you at your ease and enable you to enjoy the treatment.

If you are interested in therapeutic massage, you should tell your masseur exactly what your condition is and where your worst aches and pains are. You should also, to be on the safe side, let your doctor know that you are having massage. You should check with your doctor before signing up for any massage that includes very deep pressure or soft tissue manipulation. Your doctor may advise only light massage.

If you suffer from any of the following conditions, you should not have a massage unless your doctor gives his or her approval:
- cancer, epilepsy, HIV or AIDS
- skin infections, inflammations, bruising or recent scar tissue
- varicose veins, phlebitis or thrombosis
- undiagnosed lumps or bumps.

CASE HISTORY

John's partner Jill won a weekend at a health farm in a competition, and she suggested he go along too. As John suffered from arthritis, he was feeling rather nervous about his stay. "I imagined the place would be full of bronzed, honed bodies," he said. "But it wasn't like that at all, in fact many were in a worse state than me."

"All the treatments were optional, but down on my card was a massage. I'd never had one before, and didn't much like the idea of taking my clothes off in front of a stranger. But the masseur went out of the room while I undressed and covered myself up with towels. I told him about my arthritis, and he said he was trained to massage arthritis patients. He asked me where the inflammation was worst, and got started. After I got used to his hands on me, it started feeling wonderful, and I could actually sense my joints easing and the pain receding.

"Now I have a therapeutic massage whenever I can afford it. My doctor approves – so does Jill who says it makes me better-tempered. I think, perhaps like many men, that I had never experienced the sensation of being so cosseted before. I would probably never have thought about massage if I hadn't gone to the health farm, but massage has given me a new lease of life.

"Apart from easing the pain and inflammation, the massage helps me to calm down and relax, which I've never found easy at the best of times. When lying on that massage table, you have no choice but to relax. You can't suddenly get up and make some phone calls, for instance – and I think this 'time out' is probably doing me more good than the pills I'm taking."

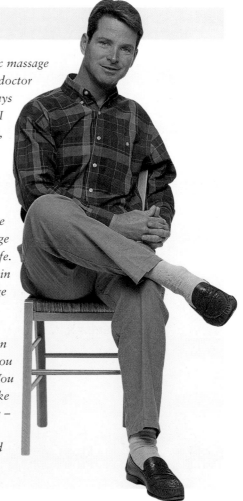

Alexander technique

The fundamental theory behind the Alexander technique is that the way in which you use your body affects how well it functions. By improving postural habits, the technique can ease the joint and muscle pain caused by arthritis.

F. Matthias Alexander, the man who developed the postural technique that bears his name, was an Australian actor who in the late nineteenth century earned his living by declaiming orations and soliloquies from the classics.

When he unaccountably lost his voice, it seemed that this might spell the end of a glittering and lucrative career for a young man who at the age of 16 had been so poor he was forced to work down a tin mine. Still only in his twenties, Alexander consulted doctor after doctor, none of whom seemed able to help, or to discover any reason for the recurring disability.

Alexander decided to help himself. With the aid of specially positioned mirrors, he watched himself rehearsing his speeches, and came to the conclusion that his loss of voice might in fact have something to do with the way in which he held his head.

Alexander observed that when he started to declaim, he had a tendency to pull his head back and downward, and he became convinced that this was the reason that he kept losing his voice.

The difficulty lay in how to stop this behaviour, as he knew that he was completely unaware of these head movements while he was reciting. Eventually, Alexander deduced that the only reason for these unnatural jerking movements was ingrained habit or, as he termed it, "use".

THE ALEXANDER TECHNIQUE AND THE NECK

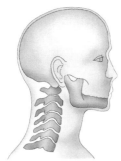

The neck connects the head and the body. When the bones of the neck align correctly, speech and swallowing mechanisms work well.

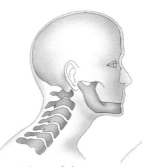

One of the most common postural problem is to push the head forward, with the result that the neck tilts permanently forward.

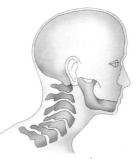

To correct a sloping neck, many people arch the neck back so that only the upper bones align correctly while the lower slope forward.

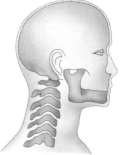

The Alexander technique re-educates the body so that the vertebrae of the neck align correctly, eliminating problems.

Alexander's discoveries

From close self-observation, Alexander concluded that it was not possible to separate mind, body and emotions, as all worked together. This concept, then revolutionary, became one of the main tenets of the Alexander philosophy.

Alexander also came to realize that whatever an individual did with one part of the body inevitably affected other areas, and that there was no such thing as an isolated body action. Through constant repetition, certain actions eventually would become ingrained, and unconscious.

This caused no problems provided that these habits were healthy ones. The difficulty arose when so many aspects of modern life – as Alexander observed in the 1920s and 1930s – predispose us to using our bodies in detrimental ways. We slump in chairs, we put too much energy into mundane tasks such as washing up, and we walk with rounded shoulders. In time, these habits become so ingrained that we cannot change them without a tremendous, conscious effort. Many poor physical habits, Alexander proposed, are initially caused by the mental or emotional problems of stress, tension and fear.

How we learn bad habits

Small children naturally walk upright but, when they go to school, according to Alexander, the combination of boredom and (then, but perhaps less now) fear that they frequently experience makes them hold their bodies tensely. Children, in addition, copy the way that adults behave and, as the majority of adults have themselves developed poor postural habits, children soon develop the same bad habits that may then remain with them for a lifetime.

Alexander maintained that many physical illnesses, including arthritis, are the result of long years of holding and using our bodies poorly. Arthritis is a good example of years of wrong usage that eventually leads to pain, disability and sometimes deformity. When this stage is reached, the only solution is to unlearn the bad habits, bring them back into conscious awareness, and teach the body new, good habits.

In order to stay well and healthy, according to Alexander, we must concentrate above all on the "use of the self" as he put it, and stay aware always of the manner in which we are sitting, standing, moving and generally conducting ourselves physically. Most people perform their day-to-day actions unconsciously, unaware that they may be damaging their bodies.

The spine's role

Alexander believed that the most important part of the body is the spine, as this is where primary control rests. Whatever happens in the spine affects the rest of the body – bones, joints, internal organs, digestion, elimination – as all other parts of the body connect to the spine directly or indirectly. In order to do its job properly, the spine must remain in its "lengthened" state. When the spine is continually shortened, such as when we slump or slouch, undue strain is put on all the limbs and organs of the body.

Find out more

What causes arthritis?   *30–37*
Alexander technique   *76–77*
Physical therapies   *116–121*

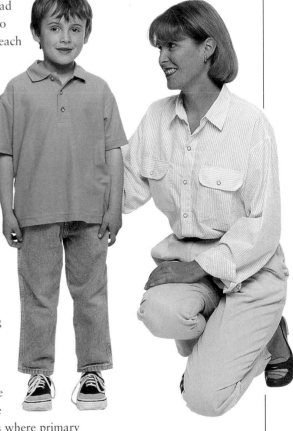

Children are not born with poor posture, but years of sitting slumped in front of a TV, or hunched over schoolwork, may throw the bones of their shoulders, neck and spine out of alignment. It is up to parents to help children "unlearn" poor practices before they become habits.

Alexander technique

How you stand greatly affects wear and tear on the spine, as well as on other joints and bones. Your teacher will help you to "feel" when your spine is correctly aligned.

Posture and health

In Alexander's view, all diseases and illnesses are manifestations of a lack of harmony in the human system, and many medical conditions have their root cause in mental or emotional stress. Stress may be held in the body for many years, maybe even a lifetime, and physical symptoms, which may be serious or even life-threatening, will eventually result.

Alexander observed that if you try to work only on the mind, without attending to the body, there is a danger that the problem will be masked rather than cured. As mental distress tends to be held and remembered in the body, close attention has to be paid to what has happened to the body to see what damage can be corrected.

Osteoarthritis is considered in mainstream medicine to be the result of years of wear and tear on the joints and, therefore, more or less inevitable. However, Alexander believed that if you use your limbs properly, you will not develop arthritis, however old you are. It is certainly true that many elderly teachers of the Alexander technique, some now in their eighties and nineties, do not suffer from osteoarthritis or bent posture, but are as upright and straight as they were in their youth.

Although the technique benefits the mind and the mental outlook, as it paves the way for a more positive approach to life, Alexander teachers work mainly on the body, and concentrate on improving posture. Once this is corrected, they believe, good health and a positive attitude will follow.

Alexander termed those people who concentrated on ends rather than means as "end-gainers", and felt that these people were the most predisposed to illness and degenerative conditions. For instance, when picking up a heavy load, you should concentrate more on how you pick it up and carry it than on reaching its ultimate destination.

An Alexander session

The Alexander technique would suit those who like the idea of a physical therapy, but who are not keen on removing all their clothes. Sessions are usually held on a one-to-one basis, but group classes are sometimes available.

You should wear loose-fitting, easy garments, such as a tracksuit and sweatshirt. Your teacher will ask you to sit, stand and lie down, and as you do so he or she will observe you closely, noting any tensions, strains and asymmetries. At your first lesson, the technique will be briefly explained to you, and you will be asked for a full medical history and questioned about your general health.

After about 15 minutes of initial consultation, you will be asked to lie on a table rather like a massage table, with your knees bent, and your head supported. This is to enable you to lie with a perfectly flat spine on the table.

The teacher will then test your muscles and joints, and ask you to sit and stand in certain positions. He or she will then demonstrate the correct Alexander way of sitting and standing. You will probably be given some simple postures to practise between consultations. As time goes on, you will begin to recognize when your body is out of alignment, and be able to give yourself the instructions for correct usage and posture.

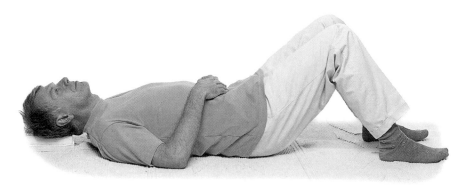

Find out more

Choosing a
    practitioner   106–107
Useful addresses   155

*Lie on a flat surface with
your feet flat on the floor,
so that your lower spine is
pushed into the surface.*

*An Alexander teacher will
help you sit and then
stand from sitting. The
tendency is to arch the
back and neck, thrusting
the head forward. Your
teacher will correct this,
perhaps by holding your
neck and spine erect.*

Learning to unlearn

Many people find Alexander lessons
enjoyable and beneficial, and begin to feel
better after just one session.

The lessons that you learn at an
Alexander session are not initially easy to
put into practice in everyday life. Years,
perhaps decades, of wrong use take time,
effort and dedication to correct. The
emphasis at Alexander lessons is always
on unlearning, rather than learning. You
have to learn to "unsit" and "unstand"
and to take your time in performing these
movements, rather than just doing them
without thought. Above all, the Alexander
technique teaches you how to perform
actions for themselves, rather than with
just the end result in mind.

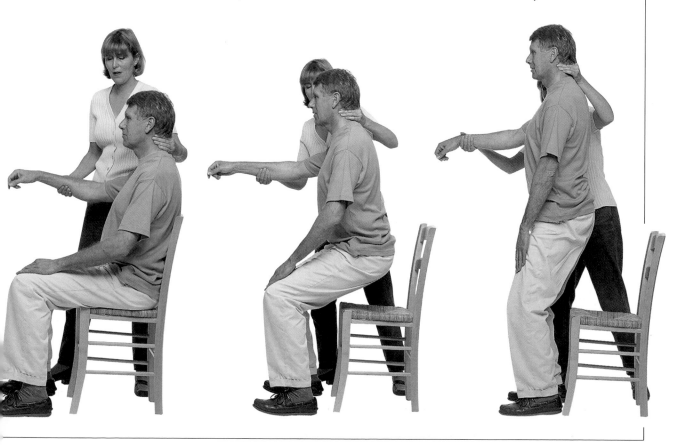

Acupuncture and acupressure

Acupuncturists treat more patients with arthritis and back pain than any other complaint. Both osteoarthritis and rheumatoid arthritis have been found to respond well to both the traditional Chinese form of the therapy and its Western form.

In patients with arthritis, acupuncturists usually find that the treatment is more successful in less severe cases, before the condition has become chronic and the degenerative changes that cause both restricted movement and severe pain are already underway.

Acupuncture cannot cure arthritis but it can alleviate the pain associated with the condition for longer and longer periods with each successive treatment. Even temporary relief from pain, without the use of medication, is a bonus for arthritis sufferers.

The word "acupuncture" comes from the Latin *acus*, meaning needle, and *punctus*, meaning to puncture or prick. Patients are treated by inserting very thin, hairlike needles into the skin at particular points. The acupuncture points lie along what are known in the Chinese tradition as meridians, or invisible energy channels. There are 14 major meridians, 12 of which are connected to particular internal organs, after which the meridian is named.

Traditional Chinese Medicine

Practitioners believe that our life force, our energy, flows along the meridians. The life force, known as *qi* or *chi* (pronounced "chee"), comprises two principal components: yin and yang. The balance of yin and yang is crucial to a well-balanced mind and healthy body. Yin, the female life force, is traditionally believed to be passive and peaceful. Yang, the male force, is thought to be aggressive and confrontational. While yin represents dark, cold, moisture and swelling, yang represents light, heat, dryness and tautness. And while yin represents rest, earth, inwardness and water, yang represents activity, heaven, expansion and fire. Any imbalance between yin and yang is considered to cause disease and disorders. This theory, of course, is completely different from those that underpin Western medicine.

Because our energy flows along the meridians, and because disease represents an imbalance of our life forces, acupuncturists seek to free, or unblock, the meridians to restore the movement of energy along the meridians. This is done by stimulating the acupuncture points.

There are up to 1,000 acupuncture points. Traditionally it was believed that there were 365, one for each day of the year. Acupuncturists in Western practices

ACUPUNCTURE NEEDLES

Acupuncture needles are usually made from stainless steel. The needles are about 2.5 cm (1 in) in length, with the same length of grip. They are solid and have a rounded end, which gently parts the flesh as it is inserted. Needles are either disposable or are rigorously sterilized between individual treatments.

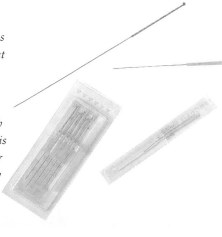

use no more than 200 points and some use fewer than this; traditional Chinese acupuncturists use a greater number of needles for longer periods of time.

Does acupuncture work?

For a Westerner, the question of whether or not you can intellectually accept the theory of acupuncture is less important than these two questions: Does it work? Is it safe? Acupuncture has been practised for thousands of years as one element of orthodox Chinese medicine. It is used to cure disease and to relieve pain. It has been used for analgesia during childbirth and surgical operations have been carried out under anaesthesia using acupuncture. This much is well documented and cannot be disputed. Clearly, acupuncture works.

How does acupuncture work?

Western experts believe that stimulation of the acupuncture points (by hairlike needles in acupuncture, by fingertip pressure in acupressure and by heat in moxibustion – see page 81) leads to the release of two sets of chemicals into the bloodstream: endorphins, the pleasure and painkilling hormones; and encephalins, which dull the senses. This results in pain relief. It is maintained that when the needle is inserted, a nerve impulse is directed to the spinal column, triggering the release of endorphins.

Other experts subscribe to the gate theory of pain. This claims that pain impulses can be regulated by a gate along the pathways of the nervous system and that certain nerve fibres, when stimulated by acupuncture or acupressure, close the gate and thus shut off the pain.

Acupuncture charts show the body's 14 main meridians and the relevant acupuncture points situated along them. The points are given Chinese names and numbers along the channels; for example, sanyinjiao or Spleen 6.

Find out more

Acupuncture	*80–81*
Shiatsu	*94–95*
Reflexology	*96–98*

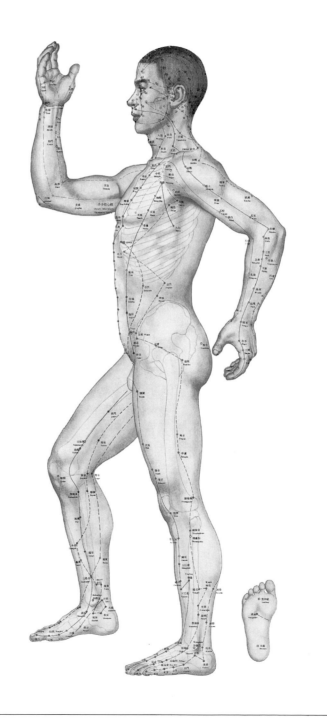

Acupuncture and acupressure

Is acupuncture safe?

Because a therapy is described as alternative, complementary or natural does not necessarily imply that it is safe. Acupuncture is generally regarded as safe, but there is one important point to observe: the practitioner should use disposable needles. Some say that sterilized needles are acceptable, but for greater safety they should be disposable and used for one patient only.

Other hazards associated with acupuncture include fainting, increased pain and pneumothorax (puncture of the lung). Although instances of these are known, they are rare.

Acupuncture is now used in orthodox pain clinics in health centres in most Western countries. Many allopathic doctors subscribe to its effectiveness, even if they cannot agree on the exact mechanisms by which it works.

The consultation

When you visit an acupuncturist for the first time, he or she will determine your general state of health by taking a detailed medical history and asking you questions about your lifestyle, diet, what sort of exercise you do, your sleep patterns and stress levels.

The acupuncturist will treat you according to the ancient rules of Chinese diagnosis. Your tongue, skin colouring and condition, your hair, posture and general air of wellbeing will all be noted, along with the sound of your breathing and your voice.

The acupuncturist will also use pulse diagnosis in order to determine how best to treat you. This enables the practitioner to gauge the state of energy in the meridians simply by taking the radial artery pulse at the wrist.

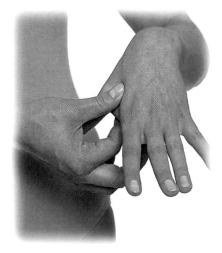

Acupressure point LI4, with pressure applied by the thumb and forefinger, is manipulated to relieve pain of all kinds. This is a good, quick remedy for minor aches and pains associated with arthritis.

There are six pulses at each wrist, making 12 in all. Each pulse represents one of the 12 main organs of the body. Taking the pulses is known as palpating. The experienced acupuncturist can diagnose many different conditions by palpating.

Once the acupuncturist has ascertained the full picture of your state of health, she or he will carefully insert needles into the acupuncture points at certain places on your body.

The insertion of needles is usually quick, painless and bloodless. They are inserted to a depth of about 6–12 mm (0.25–0.5 in) and then rotated gently between finger and thumb to stimulate energy or relieve pressure from the acupuncture point. You may experience a slight numbness or tingling sensation. The acupuncturist may use only one or two needles or up to a dozen or more. The needles are left in for anything from a few minutes to more than half an hour.

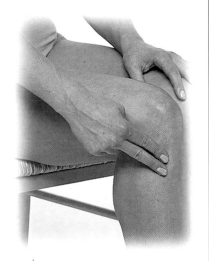

Touch is used instinctively by humans to provide comfort and relief from pain. Acupressure has developed from this instinct, using touch and pressure on a number of points all over the body to relieve specific complaints.

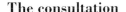

The arthritis sufferer may feel some relief from pain with one visit, but it is more likely to take several visits, maybe half a dozen, before a real benefit is perceived. It may also be that you will need to continue with acupuncture sessions for the relief of pain, as you may find that the relief does not prove to be long lasting. If you find no noticeable relief after more than seven or eight sessions, you are advised to consult another acupuncturist or to try a completely different therapy. It may be that acupuncture does not work for you.

At home

Although you cannot actually practise acupuncture on yourself, you can make use of the knowledge you gain during your visit to an acupuncturist by applying acupressure. To do this, simply massage or apply gentle pressure with your fingertips to those points that afford you the best relief in your acupuncture sessions. Ask your acupuncturist to explain how best to do this and which points to concentrate upon.

Some acupuncturists leave one or two needles in place, which enables you to twiddle the needles whenever you have serious pain. Ask your acupuncturist if this is possible in your particular case.

Finding a good practitioner

The best way to find a practitioner is to ask around and obtain the name of an acupuncturist in your local area who is well thought of. In addition, you should always check out the acupuncturist you decide upon with the appropriate governing body (in Find Out More).

Alternatively, you can ask your regular family doctor or hospital consultant to recommend one. The hospital's pain clinic may also have one or more acupuncturists available.

Find out more

Shiatsu	94–95
Choosing a practitioner	106–107
Useful addresses	155

MOXIBUSTION

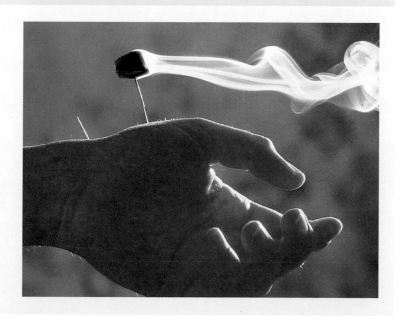

In addition to acupuncture and acupressure, the acupuncture points can be stimulated by the application of heat by a burning herb (moxibustion). Moxibustion is designed to warm the qi. The practitioner places a small cone of powdered herbs (sometimes wormwood, sometimes mugwort), known as moxa, over a point close to the skin. When the cone becomes hot, it is removed and then the process is repeated, sometimes several times, until the practitioner decides the desired effect has been achieved. Moxibustion is usually applied when and where acupuncture alone proves ineffective.

Herbal medicine

Before laboratory-made drugs, nearly all medicines in all cultures were herbal remedies made from plants and plant extracts, and this remains so in some developing countries.

The blend of water and natural plant materials can combine to make herbal medicine both effective and soothing for arthritis sufferers.

Although Western scientific medicine is making fast inroads in countries such as India and China, it is still the case that 85 per cent of the population in both countries rely on traditional herbal remedies and treatment.

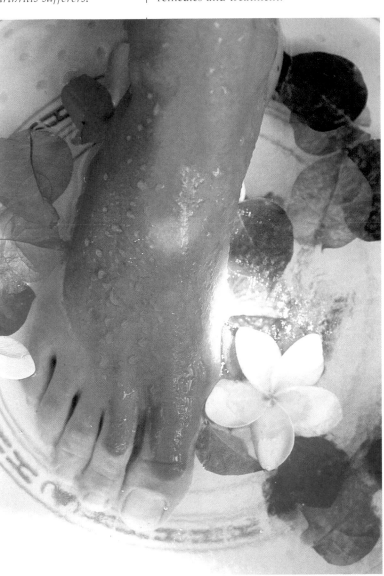

The paradox is that while Eastern countries are excitedly adopting Western medical methods, an increasing number of Westerners are turning back to herbal remedies. Although many laboratory-produced drugs owe their origins to herbal components, natural, traditional herbal remedies and the ancient skills of herbalism are now making a significant comeback.

Herbalism is an ancient art with a modern twist. Whereas the herbalists of old relied mainly on folklore handed down from one generation to another, modern herbal practitioners have to undergo rigorous training at a recognized school of herbal medicine, and their training includes working with Oriental as well as Western herbs. Because of this they have a far wider choice of treatments than practitioners in earlier times. Now that there are thousands of therapeutic herbs available to modern therapists, almost any ailment can be treated with a specific herb or combination of herbs.

Many ancient herbal remedies have now been evaluated in clinical trials at leading teaching hospitals so that, at last, we can find out why and how these ancient treatments work.

If you are interested in using herbal remedies for arthritis, it is important that you consult with your regular doctor first. Unlike some of the other complementary therapies, herbalism is not always compatible with orthodox drugs. Some herbal treatments are strong, and some can exert a negative as well as a positive effect. Some herbs clash with some of the ingredients in orthodox medication.

Herbs work quite differently from pharmaceutical drugs. Fundamental to the herbalist's view is that plants are used to restore balance and harmony to the whole body, rather than simply to treat symptoms. Because the whole plant, rather than its isolated chemicals, are used, there is less risk of overdose or adverse side-effects.

A visit to a herbal clinic is usually a more interesting experience than visiting a conventional doctor's surgery. As with other forms of complementary medicine, the herbalist will take a full case history,

asking about your medical history, your general lifestyle, diet, exercise routine, work, and personal stresses.

The chosen herbal remedy may be combined with a diet created specially for you, some beneficial exercises and advice on ways to reduce stress. As with other complementary treatments, modern herbal medicine is a holistic treatment.

Herbal treatments can be prescribed in the form of pills, teas, tisanes or tinctures, ointments, infusions, drops, suppositories, enemas, herbal baths, poultices or syrups. You may be prescribed a mixture of different herbal essences which you burn and then inhale.

CASE HISTORY

Anita, 58, had suffered pain and stiffness in her knees for the past four years. The problem was gradually getting worse, and she decided to see a herbalist after watching a television programme on the subject.

"The office where I work is on the fifth floor, and there is no lift. I noticed that climbing stairs made my condition worse, and that gardening, which I enjoy, was getting increasingly difficult to do. I felt that a herbalist might take more trouble than an ordinary doctor. I was taking pills to alleviate the stiffness, but, as I didn't want to take drugs long-term, this was another reason for trying an alternative.

The herbalist asked about my diet, and told me I was slightly overweight, which I of course knew anyway.

The consultation was very thorough. The herbalist X-rayed my knees, took my blood pressure, examined my tongue

and took my pulse. He diagnosed osteoarthritis, resulting from poor circulation and my being overweight. Too much standing and living in a damp, cold country had made the condition worse, he said. I had actually noticed that the arthritis improved when on holiday in Spain.

The herbal treatments he prescribed were to drain the tissues of accumulated waste, stimulate circulation and reduce inflammation. The prescription he gave me was complicated, and involved infusions, tinctures, poultices and footbaths. He also recommended swimming and brisk walking, and put me on a wholefood diet.

Both the consultation and the treatment were extremely pleasant experiences and, as well as dramatic improvement of the stiffness, I feel so much better in myself."

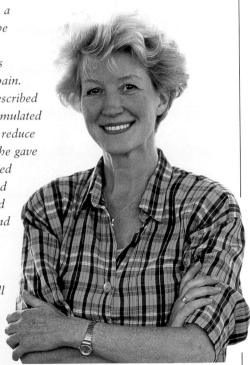

Herbal medicine

Herbal treatments tend to be slower-acting than laboratory drugs, and, as they have a gentler action, are useful for chronic complaints. In fact, for a number of intractable conditions, such as eczema and asthma, herbal medicine is superseding orthodox treatment.

Seeking treatment

You can buy herbal treatments from high-street pharmacies, but herbal medicine for a serious condition such as arthritis should not be regarded as a self-help treatment. Herbal treatments can be very complicated, and should be administered by a fully trained medical herbalist. Word of mouth recommendation is the best way to choose a practitioner, but if this is not possible ask their governing body for a list of qualified herbalists in your area. Even if you do have a personal recommendation, you should check your

chosen herbalist's qualifications with the governing body.

As with other treatments for arthritis, whether orthodox or complementary, nothing can guarantee a cure or permanent remission from the condition.

During a consultation

The herbalist will consider not only the symptoms which are causing your problem, but your whole body. Herbs may be prescribed to stimulate or relax bodily functions (such as digestion or circulation), or to increase energy levels. You will be given suggestions on diet, such as increasing your intake of wholefoods and cutting down on tea, coffee and cola. The aim is to encourage the body to heal itself, rather than to suppress symptoms.

British herbalist Michael McIntyre says: "Toxic elements which have

Basic herbal remedies are easy to make at home. Taking a few minutes out of a busy day just to prepare a herbal tea can be relaxing and therapeutic in itself.

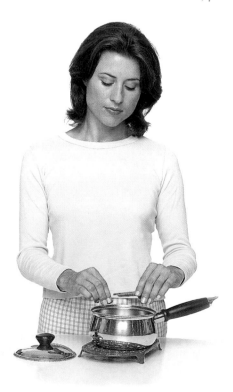
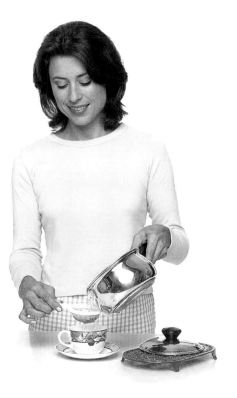

accumulated over many years may be gently released using deep-acting herbs. We would also use specific herbs to help the organs of elimination, such as the liver and kidneys, to work properly again. This is especially important nowadays, as so many patients who come to us have been taking a variety of highly potent and dangerously toxic drugs for years."

Herbs are not always safe

- If you experience side-effects, stop taking the remedy
- Do not exceed the stated dose
- Do not take for prolonged periods as it is not known whether or not it is safe to do so
- Do not pick from the wild
- Do not buy from abroad.

Find out more

Choosing a practitioner	*106–107*
Diet	*142–147*
Useful organizations	*155*

SOME HERBAL REMEDIES

The following herbs have been found to be useful in the treatment of arthritis:

MEADOWSWEET	Meadowsweet is the herb most often prescribed for arthritis. It contains salicylic (aspirin-like) glycosides and has a potent anti-inflammatory action
DEVIL'S CLAW	Devil's claw is also an anti-inflammatory, and in scientific tests has been compared favourably with phenylbutazone, a commonly prescribed mainstream anti-inflammatory drug
BURDOCK	Burdock may be used to deep-cleanse the tissues
CELERY SEED	Celery seed stimulates the elimination of uric acid and is therefore especially useful in treating gout
CORNSILK	Cornsilk strengthens the kidneys
HORSETAIL	Horsetail strengthens the kidneys
NETTLE	This common weed improves circulation and also helps to rid the body of excess harmful acids
SARSAPARILLA	Sarsaparilla detoxifies the body
PRICKLY ASH	Prickly ash aids circulation

Your herbalist may also use Chinese herbs such as *Achyranthes* (for getting rid of "dampness" in the joints), angelica and large-leaf gentian.

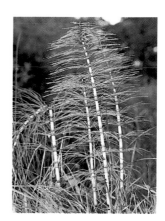

Horsetail has long been associated with the relief of kidney complaints.

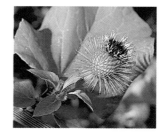

Burdock has large, heart-shaped leaves and purple flowers. It is appreciated for its tissue-cleansing properties.

Homeopathy

Homeopathic medicine is based on the theory that "like cures like" and it has been used for over two hundred years. For example, a hot, tender, swollen joint that is relieved by cold applications would be treated with Apis, made from bees, because the symptoms are similar to those of a bee sting.

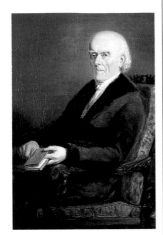

Samuel Hahnemann (1755–1843), a German doctor, is the founder of homeopathy. He discovered that when a so-called "similar" substance was used to a disease – similar in its ability to produce a symptom and therefore able to stimulate the body's own healing system into stopping the symptom – people were healed gently, and permanently.

Hahnemann's careful observations of conventional medicine showed him that it was based on the law of opposites. In other words, doctors prescribed a medicine to make the body go into the opposite mode. For example, a person with a runny nose would take a medicine to stop their nose running. A homeopath, on the other hand, would administer a substance which in a healthy person would produce a runny nose – and the sufferer would be cured.

Homeopathic remedies, the name given to the medicines used, are made from plants, minerals, animals and some diseased matter. They go through a process of dilution and shaking known as potentization, through which the substance's healing power is released and all harmful, toxic qualities are eliminated. The remedy acts as a stimulant for the body to heal itself and restore a balance of health. All such remedies are readily available from homeopaths, from homeopathic pharmacies, and from increasing numbers of high-street pharmacies.

As homeopathy is a holistic form of healing, treating mind and body equally, there are no remedies for ailments, but rather for people who suffer particular symptoms in their own individual way. Their individuality is what leads the homeopath to identify the correct remedy. When prescribing treatments, homeopaths take into account the patient's state of mind, outlook, personality and general behaviour as well as the illness itself. As with most other forms of complementary treatment, homeopathy is intended to stimulate the body's own self-healing mechanism and to work without adverse side-effects.

Central to the concept of homeopathy is that the smaller the dose, the more potent it becomes. This idea, which conflicts with conventional medical belief, has proved one of the most difficult stumbling blocks in homeopathy's long struggle for acceptance by the mainstream medical profession.

The amount of "active ingredient" in homeopathic medicine is that which produces a curative effect without toxic or adverse side-effects. Thus, homeopathy is never harmful. However, as it is such a delicate treatment, its effects can be negated by strong drugs, foods or smells.

Many orthodox doctors consider that homeopathic remedies are no more than placebo, as they contain no discernible active ingredients. However, homeopathy is becoming more popular, and it is now not unusual to find that at least one doctor in a health centre is also a qualified homeopath.

Homeopathic remedies can work well with animals. In particular, homeopathy has had great success with racehorses which, since they are valuable animals with delicate systems, have to be given the gentlest, most effective treatment available, without the risk of damaging side-effects. This tends to undermine detractors who claim that homeopathic remedies work only on the mind.

Although many homeopathic remedies can now be bought over the counter from high-street chemists, anyone suffering from a chronic condition such as arthritis would be well advised to consult a qualified homeopath. As many homeopathic doctors are also qualified in orthodox medicine, they can understand the arthritis from both points of view, and can recommend mainstream treatments if they feel that these are required.

Like other complementary therapies, homeopathy cannot treat structural damage that requires surgery. If you need a hip replacement, for example, homeopathy cannot help. It cannot repair worn-out joints or correct bone deformities. However, the appropriate homeopathic remedies can speed up the healing process after surgery. They can also work as preventative treatment, and thus guard against future damage and deformity which might be caused by chronic arthritis.

QUESTIONS YOUR HOMEOPATH MAY ASK

ARE YOUR SYMPTOMS AFFECTED BY MOVEMENT?	Symptoms that seem to be better when you are still may require a different remedy from a condition that is improved with movement.
HOW SUDDEN WAS THE ONSET OF SYMPTOMS?	Your homeopath will need to know whether your symptoms have come on suddenly, perhaps violently, or whether the symptoms have been gradually getting worse over a certain period of time.
AT WHAT TIME OF DAY OR NIGHT ARE YOUR SYMPTOMS AT THEIR WORST?	The time at which symptoms are worst is an important factor in making a homeopathic diagnosis. A remedy that would be prescribed for a pain that is worse in the evening would not necessarily be suitable for symptoms that reach their peak in the morning.
HOW DO CHANGES IN TEMPERATURE AFFECT YOUR SYMPTOMS?	In homeopathy the effect of heat or cold is very important in deciding the right remedy. A pain that is worse when you are cold is likely to require different treatment from one that is worse when you are hot.
DID ANY SPECIAL FACTORS PROVOKE THE ONSET OF SYMPTOMS?	It is important for your homeopath to know if your symptoms followed a significant event. This may be a sudden emotional shock such as a bereavement, or a more mundane occurrence such as exposure to cold or damp.
WHAT KIND OF PERSONALITY DO YOU HAVE?	The type of person you are – withdrawn or extrovert, cautious or impulsive, for example – is a factor in determining the best treatment for you, so two people with similar symptoms are likely to be prescribed different remedies.
HOW IS YOUR THIRST?	It may be significant to the diagnosis whether you are particularly thirsty or if you crave hot or cold drinks.

Homeopathy

At the initial consultation, you will be asked detailed questions about your arthritis. You will also be asked to provide your medical history from the time of your mother's pregnancy onwards, including any childhood illnesses, and you will be asked about your lifestyle, likes and dislikes in life and the regularity of your bodily functions. You may also be asked about your work and your interests. Be sure to tell your homeopath if you are taking or have recently been taking any orthodox drugs.

At the end of the consultation you will be prescribed a suitable remedy or group of remedies which you can obtain from a homeopathic pharmacy. Hahnemann also placed great emphasis on nutrition, and you will probably be given guidance and advice on this, so as to minimise your symptoms and possible future flare-ups of your arthritis.

There are more than 2,000 homeopathic remedies in the *Materia Medica*, the homeopath's main reference book. The homeopath may also use a repertory, an index of symptoms, which may be computerized. Most of the remedies are derived from plants and minerals, but some come from animal or human tissues or secretions. A few are derived from micro-organisms that multiply during disease processes and a few have been developed from modern drugs. Most remedies are given Latin names, or abbreviations of these. Such names may make them sound rather mysterious, but a good homeopath will be able to explain them to you.

Most modern homeopathic remedies come in the form of lactose pills impregnated with a solution of the remedy. The pills are simply dissolved on the tongue: they have no particular taste.

Some remedies are sold in solution form in small glass phials with screw tops, and a few are available as ointments.

In many countries, homeopathic remedies are available under health insurance schemes, provided that they are prescribed by a qualified physician. In the United Kingdom, for example, they are available on the National Health Service if they have been prescribed by a doctor. The National Health Service also runs five homeopathic hospitals; despite their names, these hospitals promote a range of complementary therapies, not only homeopathy.

While taking homeopathic remedies, you may be advised to modify your lifestyle, as experience has shown that the remedies do not mix well with some substances. The efficacy of the remedies may be reduced or negated if, at the same time, you are smoking, drinking alcohol or a lot of tea, coffee or colas. You should avoid brushing your teeth for 15 minutes before and after taking a remedy. You may be asked to avoid highly perfumed toiletries, strong smelling household cleaners, and some essential oils. Some aromatherapy oils also clash with homeopathic treatments.

Homeopathic remedies are unlikely to interfere with any orthodox drugs you may be taking, although many of these, such as steroids, sleeping pills and anti-histamines, will block the effects of homeopathic remedies, making them a waste of money.

If you would like to stop taking your orthodox drugs before trying a homeopathic approach, consult your doctor first and ensure that this will not endanger your health. Never suddenly stop a course of orthodox treatment without consulting your doctor.

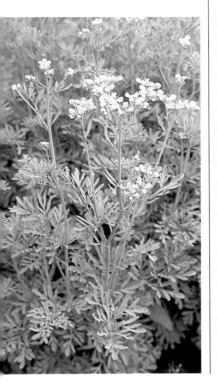

Ruta graveolens *is the homeopathic remedy which is based on the garden herb common rue.*

Find out more

Choosing a
practitioner   106–107

SOME SUITABLE HOMEOPATHIC REMEDIES

There are a number of remedies that are effective in treating arthritis. Homeopaths believe in prescribing for the individual's constitution rather than for the condition. What works for one person may not for another, so a consultation is necessary.

RHUS TOX (RHUS TOXICODENDRON OR POISON IVY)	Rhus tox is the most commonly indicated homeopathic remedy for arthritis and rheumatism that get better with the application of heat and worse after sitting for long periods. Patients who feel stiff on rising, and for whom continuous and sustained movement gives relief, would benefit from this remedy.
BRYONIA (WHITE COMMON BRYONY OR OLD MEN'S BEARD)	Bryonia is useful for very painful joint conditions that are made worse by the least movement, but improve after rest and immobilization.
RUTA (RUE)	Ruta is a useful general remedy for complaints that affect the tendons and ligaments such as tennis elbow.
CALC. PHOS (CALCIUM PHOSPHATE)	Calc. phos. is a useful general remedy for arthritis of the hands.
CALC. CARB. (CALCAREA CARBONICA, OYSTERSHELL)	Calc. carb. is particularly useful in the treatment of osteoarthritis.
ARS. ALB (WHITE ARSENIC)	Although potentially lethal in the wrong hands, used homeopathically arsenic can in fact bring relief, particularly to those whose symptoms are markedly worse at night and improve with heat.
PULSATILLA (WINDFLOWER)	A commonly prescribed homeopathic remedy with many uses, this is used to relieve symptoms which are made worse by heat and improve in the open air.
APIS (BEE STING)	This homeopathic remedy is useful for the sudden onsets or flare ups of hot, swollen, tender joints, which are relieved by cold application, that often occur with some types of arthritis.

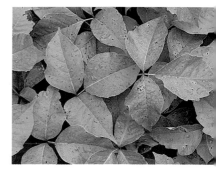

Rhus tox, *poison ivy, is the treatment for many forms of arthritis.*

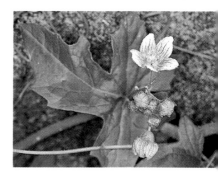

White bryony is used to treat joint problems, including arthritis.

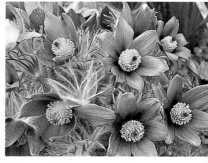

The windflower is used in the homeopathic remedy known as Pulsatilla.

Osteopathy

*O*ne of the skills of treating pain by correcting bone and joint problems through expert manipulation is known as osteopathy. It is generally accepted by mainstream medicine.

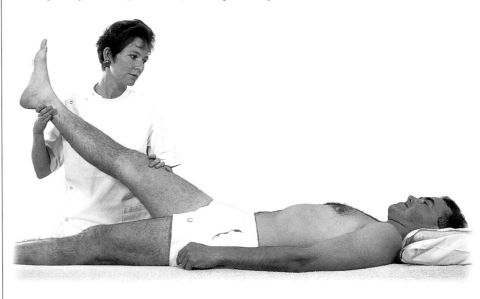

A trained osteopath will examine your skeletal system and its muscles and connecting tissues before deciding on the appropriate treatment.

There are a family of manipulative techniques, which includes osteopathy, chiropractic and orthopaedic medicine. People have manipulated joints to help them function smoothly for centuries, but osteopathy in its modern form was developed by Andrew Still, a doctor in the American Civil War.

Dr Still became convinced that the spine was the source of good health and that if you were able to heal the spine, the rest of the body would respond positively. He believed that such conditions as vertebrae out of alignment and malfunctioning joints impeded the circulation of the blood and affected the workings of the nervous system, which prevented the body from fighting disease. Still first tried manipulating joints in the interest of health in 1874. It took nearly 100 years for osteopathy to become accepted as a serious scientific discipline for disorders involving bones and joints.

Osteopaths rely on their manipulative abilities to bring relief of pain and to restore mobility to stiff and painful joints. In the USA, osteopaths have the full status of doctors and are often accepted by the mainstream medical profession. They can refer patients to other specialists, and some practise surgery. In other Western countries, osteopaths have not acquired this status.

Osteopathy is similar to chiropractic and both therapies can treat identical conditions using similar techniques; however, there are some differences between the two therapies. Osteopaths do more soft-tissue work both by superficial massage and by deep massage than chiropractors, and they mobilize the joints by traction or articulation. This means that they put the joints through their full range of movement passively, for a more specific thrust than might be given by a chiropractor.

Treating arthritis

Osteopathy is suitable for osteoarthritis and wear-and-tear conditions of the spine, but less so for rheumatoid arthritis and other forms of inflammatory arthritis. Osteopaths can often help to relieve the symptoms of arthritis, but as with any doctor they cannot cure the condition. For sufferers of severe arthritis, instant relief from pain and stiffness is blissful, but with time, the joints will stiffen again. Osteopathy does not reduce inflammation, nor will it prevent waste matter accumulating in joints.

Although osteopathy is no longer considered an alternative treatment, some orthodox doctors remain sceptical of the treatment. They believe that arthritis is characterized by periods of remission and of acute or chronic pain, so it is difficult to determine whether osteopathy treatment has helped or whether the illness simply went into remission. Some orthodox doctors – and some patients – believe that osteopathy can be dangerous.

However, it is one of the safer forms of physical treatment for arthritis, provided that the therapist is properly qualified.

Osteopaths usually work in well-equipped clinics and take a detailed case history, which includes asking you about your medical history and current lifestyle. Treatment sessions generally last for about an hour, and up to six treatments will usually be indicated, depending upon the severity of your arthritis.

For arthritis sufferers, the main benefit of osteopathy comes from manipulating the joints in the skeleton, and some bones may even alter their position with successive treatments. Osteopaths believe that the secret of their treatment is interspersing manipulative therapy with periods of rest to give the body its best chance of healing itself. After your treatment, you will be given advice on how best to rest your joints. There are no adverse side-effects and, if the treatment has worked efficiently, you should feel better.

Find out more

| Chiropractic | 92–93 |
| Choosing a practitioner | 106–107 |

CASE HISTORY

Bill started to experience pain in his joints in his mid-40s. He had always been athletic, had played football and now squash. Bill booked a session with the osteopath attached to the health centre where he played.

"The osteo first took a case history, then asked me to undress down to my underpants and to lie down on the floor. He started pressing on my joints, asking me to tell him where the pain was. I was horrified when he diagnosed arthritis, as I thought my keep-fit activities would have prevented it. But he reckoned it was probably caused by wear and tear when playing football.

"He started manipulating the sore areas, and the relief was immediate. The first session lasted 45 minutes, and the subsequent ones 20 to 30 minutes. The treatment was rough and strong, and suited me. It has enabled me to keep the arthritis at bay, and occasionally I have a maintenance session. The best thing for me is not relying on drugs."

Chiropractic

Chiropractic is similar to osteopathy and orthopaedic medicine in that it alleviates pain by manipulating the joints. There are minor differences in the techniques used to manipulate the joints. Chiropractors may use X-rays to help diagnose various problems, whereas osteopaths rely on their knowledge of the human body to actually feel where there is dysfunction and immobility.

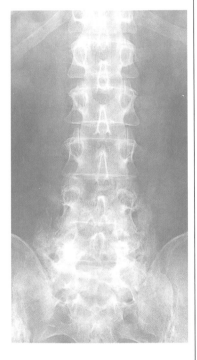

This X-ray provides a clear image of the vertebrae in the lower spinal cord of an older man. A chiropractor uses X-rays similar to this one to help diagnose a disorder. In particular, he will look for any misalignment in the vertebrae.

Chiropractors believe that using X-rays makes diagnosis more accurate and enables them to go straight to the problem. This may be reassuring to the arthritis sufferer, as it means there is less risk of manipulating – or over-manipulating – immobile joints. Your choice between the two disciplines depends on whether or not you are happy with X-rays. If you are concerned about the effect of radiation, you may decide that you would prefer osteopathy.

The first chiropractic treatment in its modern sense took place in 1895, in Davenport, Iowa, and soon became phenomenally popular. Its inventor was Daniel David Palmer, a Canadian businessman and adventurer who became interested first in magnetic healing, a popular treatment at that time. Palmer became a healer, using the "laying on of hands", and he soon became intrigued with discovering the cause of disease.

Palmer's research led him to believe that there was a close association between the vertebrae in the back and disease of all kinds. He knew that manipulation had been practised by the ancient Egyptians, and he claimed to have rediscovered the practice and brought it into modern use. Palmer also investigated the new science of osteopathy, but he formulated his own ideas about the role of the spine in relation to health.

After an initial success in treating deafness by manipulation of the spine,

Palmer established a small practice in the new discipline. However, Palmer was tried, convicted and imprisoned for practising medicine without a certificate in Scott County, Iowa, in 1906. After that, hundreds of chiropractors faced fines and jail sentences for practising medicine without a licence, and this continued in America until the 1960s.

Chiropractic became increasingly popular with the general public, and the discipline managed to thrive despite the fact that it was regarded as rather unscientific. In part, chiropractic owed its success to the fact that chiropractors were performing what came to be known as bloodless surgery, in the days when surgery was a very painful and risky – even fatal – business. Another reason for the success of chiropractic was that patients often felt better immediately after treatment. There were not usually any adverse side-effects, which can be one of the negative aspects of taking orthodox drugs and undergoing surgery.

Who can benefit?

In simple terms, a chiropractor restores normal movement to a joint that has developed some type of abnormality, so dysfunctional movement of muscles and joints will generally respond to chiropractic treatment.

Chiropractic may be indicated when the body is unable to heal itself after a bone and joint injury. It is best used for pain and disorders before the body has become irreversibly diseased.

Chiropractors look for what they term subluxations – misaligned and biochemically dysfunctioning vertebrae – and other joints that may be preventing normal functioning. As chiropractic can influence the nerve impulses that regulate beta-endorphins, the body's own natural painkillers, chiropractic treatments can work as a powerful painkiller, even when the arthritis has progressed too far for the joints to be restored to full mobility.

Very painful arthritis can be helped with chiropractic adjustment, which will encourage the body's own healing mechanisms to start working again. However, chiropractic cannot reverse or treat severe arthritis where deformity and disability already exist.

The type of arthritis or rheumatism most likely to respond positively to chiropractic is that in which the disease is mainly of neuro-muscular or vascular origin, affecting the spine and limbs. Inflammatory types are less likely to be treated by chiropractic.

How chiropractic works

According to chiropractors, the therapy works on three levels. The first is the mechanical and anatomical, which restores movement by improving functions through a variety of spinal manipulation and joint mobilization techniques. The second level is that of pain relief. The third is the mental and emotional level, and here the chiropractor practises the healing touch.

Your first visit to a chiropractor will involve the practitioner taking a detailed medical history and details of your lifestyle, followed by an assessment of your condition by expert touch and feel. Before starting any kind of treatment, the practitioner will decide whether or not chiropractic is appropriate for your condition. If so, the next step may be taking X-rays.

Chiropractic involves pushing, pulling and levering muscle against bone. The number of sessions will depend on the severity of the problem. As with osteopathy, you will feel the treatment, and you may experience some moments of pain – but it should not be extremely painful. It is important to ensure that the chiropractor is fully qualified, and has a clear understanding of the exact nature of your particular condition.

Find out more

Osteopathy	90–91
Choosing a practitioner	106–107

A chiropractor uses a number of separate techniques to manipulate the spine. You may hear the bones click during the therapy.

Shiatsu

The Japanese word shiatsu literally means "finger pressure". However, the shiatsu practitioner uses not only fingers, but also hands, thumbs, elbows and even knees or feet to achieve the desired depth and strength of massage.

The pressure provided by a shiatsu massage should produce a sensation somewhere between pain and pleasure.

This system of fingertip massage bears some similarities to acupressure – both are based on pressure points along meridian lines associated with the function of the vital organs. Like acupressure, shiatsu is designed to stimulate the body's own energy levels (*ki* in Japanese); however, instead of using the stimulation of energy to relieve pain, shiatsu places the emphasis on freeing or unblocking the energy channels to promote overall health. In other words, it lays emphasis on the prevention of disease rather than on treating specific symptoms.

In Japan, shiatsu is considered to be an effective means of early diagnosis as well as a means of disease prevention. Many people attend regular shiatsu treatments, as often as once a week.

Shiatsu is believed to benefit the body, mind, emotions and spirit, all at the same time. Its particular strengths lie in stimulating the body's immune system, which is invaluable in the treatment of arthritis and a variety of other disorders that have pain as a common feature.

The depth and strength of massage practised in shiatsu has the effect of improving the circulation and flow of lymphatic fluid, working on the nervous system, helping to release toxins and deep-seated tension from the muscles and stimulating the hormone system.

Shiatsu techniques have been known in Japan for many hundreds of years, but became popular in the West much more recently. Shiatsu was introduced to the United Kingdom in the late 1970s, and the Shiatsu Society was formed in 1981.

The consultation

The first shiatsu session usually begins with the practitioner taking a detailed medical and life history from you. Shiatsu affects all levels of your being – physical, emotional, psychological and spiritual. Treatment is attuned to your personal health and character. Your practitioner is likely to ask about your diet, what exercise you take and some queries about your current lifestyle; he or she may advise you on how to alter your regimes with a view to improving your condition.

As in acupuncture, the therapist will take your pulses, of which there are six at each wrist, each associated with a vital organ of the body. Taking the pulses helps the practitioner to diagnose and treat many different conditions.

The treatment, not unlike a massage, involves pressure being applied in many different ways, and a series of different movements may be executed over a part of the body, rather than over one particular pressure point. Sometimes the pad of the thumb is used, sometimes the

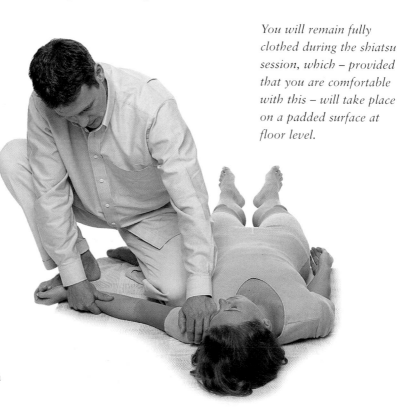

fingers, sometimes the palm or the heel of the hand. The practitioner may also use the elbow or perhaps a forearm or knee.

How hard the shiatsu practitioner applies pressure depends on many factors, including where it is to be applied, how you react and whether you require a stimulating or a sedating effect. Pressure is usually applied for a few seconds at a time, sometimes longer, and may be repeated several times at each spot. A session lasts for about an hour.

The shiatsu session is usually carried out on the floor, but if it is not possible for you to have the treatment in this position, your practitioner will still be able to treat you. The Shiatsu Society of Great Britain offers the following guidelines before you attend a consultation:

• Take a light meal at least one hour before your session. It is best not to eat heavy meals or drink alcohol on the day of your treatment.
• Do not take a long hot bath on the day of treatment.
• For the treatment itself, wear loose clothing, preferably cotton, such as a tracksuit or jogging suit.
• Have with you details of your current medical diagnosis and a record of any medication you may be taking.
• Inform your practitioner in advance if you are pregnant or if you have recently undergone any major procedure such as surgery or radiotherapy.

At home

After a shiatsu treatment, you will probably feel invigorated yet relaxed at the same time. Do not be surprised if you feel little improvement after just one treatment, as shiatsu normally takes a number of sessions to achieve an effect.

The duration and frequency of treatment will vary from person to person and with the degree of severity your arthritis has reached. You may experience headache or mild flulike symptoms for a day or so, but these are the result of the body's efforts to eliminate toxins and should be regarded as a positive sign.

Shiatsu initially developed as a home treatment, and the techniques have been handed down from one generation to the next. It is possible, therefore, to learn how to apply finger pressure yourself and to do some of the techniques at home.

Arthritis sufferers may also benefit from a related technique, known as *do-in*, which translated literally means "self-stimulation". This is a form of self-acupressure massage of muscles and points that also includes movement, stretching and breathing exercises.

You will remain fully clothed during the shiatsu session, which – provided that you are comfortable with this – will take place on a padded surface at floor level.

Reflexology

*R*eflexology is becoming increasingly well known for its ability to boost energy levels, promote a sense of wellbeing and alleviate pain. It is a therapy that is likely to be beneficial for many people suffering with arthritis.

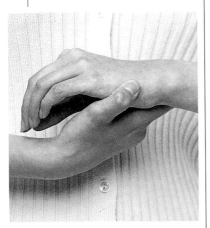

Although most reflexologists work on a patient's feet, using the corresponding pressure points on the hands is generally more convenient for self-treatment.

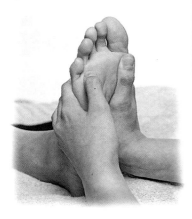

The foot is the site of the numerous pressure points used by reflexologists to stimulate a patient's healing properties.

Like acupuncture and acupressure, reflexology is based on similar principles of a life force flowing through the body along energy channels. However, in reflexology the terminal points, or reflex areas, of the energy channels lie in the feet and hands; in acupuncture, the terminal points are located all over the body. The reflexologist does not use needles to stimulate the points, only pressure; the acupuncturist uses needles. (Acupressure follows the locations of the points used in acupuncture, but applies pressure to the points rather than using needles.)

Reflexology has developed along the basic concept that every part of the body is connected to the pathways that end in reflex areas on the feet and hands. Tension or congestion in any part of the body is mirrored in the corresponding reflex areas on the feet or hands. By applying controlled pressure over these reflexes in a precise and systematic way, the reflexologist stimulates the client's body to achieve its own natural state of wholeness and good health.

The body has a great ability to heal itself. Following illness, stress and disease, the body is in a state of imbalance, with vital energy pathways blocked, which prevent it from functioning properly. Reflexologists aim to unblock these pathways, and treating the whole foot can have a deeply relaxing and healing effect on the whole body.

The practice of stimulating the body's own healing properties by using pressure points on the feet is not new. Reflexology has been practised for thousands of years, in one form or another, in different cultures around the world. For example, there is evidence that it was known over 5,000 years ago in China and 4,000 years ago in Egypt. The practice spread to Europe sometime between the fifth and ninth centuries, and forms of pressure point therapy are known to have been used in the Middle Ages.

Modern times

Modern reflexology has its roots in medical and neurological studies carried out in the United Kingdom and Germany in the 1890s. Thus the tradition of pressure-point therapy converged with new discoveries regarding zone therapy and the effects of massage on the sympathetic nervous system.

Further support was provided by Dr William Fitzgerald, an American ear, nose and throat specialist, at the turn of the nineteenth century and promoted by him from 1913. Dr Fitzgerald found that when certain points on the feet were pressed, an anaesthetic effect was induced in specific parts of the body. Through experimentation in applying pressure to different areas of the feet, either with his hands or with special instruments, he evolved a system that he named zone therapy. Reflexology, or reflex zone therapy as it was sometimes known, became popular in the USA in the 1930s and was introduced to the United Kingdom in the 1960s.

One of the underlying theories of modern reflexology is that as our ancestors walked and ran barefoot over uneven ground, the nerve endings and reflex areas on their feet were constantly being massaged and stimulated. But nowadays, we spend much of our time sitting down, and when we do walk it is usually on hard, flat surfaces, wearing thick-soled shoes to cushion our feet; consequently, they are no longer massaged and stimulated.

When women wear high heels, the balance of weight on the soles of the feet is altered, putting extra pressure on some areas and failing to stimulate others.

Who can benefit?

While reflexology cannot cure arthritis, it can alleviate chronic pain and raise your energy levels. It is used not so much for cure of disease but for easing fatigue and pain. For this reason, it works well in conjunction with other treatments, either with other complementary therapies or with conventional medicine. Many people who are taking prescribed drugs or other medical treatments find that reflexology reduces or eliminates side-effects, thus enhancing the benefits of orthodox medicine. After surgery, reflexology helps to stimulate the healing process.

One of the most interesting aspects of reflexology in the treatment of arthritis is that some practitioners believe that they can detect crystalline deposits of calcium or uric acid. If this is so, sufferers of gout could particularly benefit from a course of reflexology. However, other practitioners maintain that the deposits they feel are composed of a build-up of lactic acid.

The consultation

The reflexologist will take a detailed medical and life history from you during your first visit. He or she will then examine your feet, noting their general appearance, temperature and colour. Before treatment begins, the reflexologist will apply talcum powder to facilitate a smooth and even movement of his or her hands over the surface of your feet.

In the course of the treatment the reflexologist will exert thumb pressure of varying strengths over the pressure points of the feet, concentrating on any tender areas. These tender areas indicate those parts of the body that are out of balance. Sessions usually last for about 50 minutes and may be weekly to start with, then at intervals of two or three weeks.

During treatment, the body experiences a process of detoxification. This may later manifest itself in what could be called the side-effects of reflexology. These include aching joints, diarrhoea, increased need to urinate, feeling a little flu-ish and feeling cold. If any of these symptoms do occur, they should be regarded as a good sign, showing that the body is ridding itself of impurities and toxins. In any case, they will not last for long.

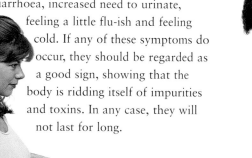
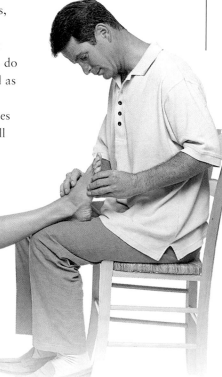

For a typical reflexology treatment you sit or lie in a comfortable, reclining position, with your feet raised and shoes and socks removed.

Reflexology

Reflexology points
Each area of the foot corresponds to a specific organ or part of the body. Where relevant (for the two lungs or the two kidneys, for example), the right foot relates to the right side of the body and the left foot to the left side.

1 *Brain/top of head*
2 *Sinuses/brain/top of head*
3 *Side of brain as well as head/neck*
4 *Pituitary gland*
5 *Spine*
6 *Neck/throat/thyroid gland*
7 *Parathyroid*
8 *Thyroid gland*

9 *Trachea*
10 *Eye*
11 *Eustachian tube*
12 *Ear*
13 *Shoulder*
14 *Lung*
15 *Heart*
16 *Solar plexus*
17 *Stomach*
18 *Pancreas*
19 *Kidney*
20 *Liver*
21 *Gall bladder*
22 *Spleen*
23 *Ascending colon*
24 *Descending colon*
25 *Small intestine*
26 *Bladder*
27 *Sciatic nerve*
28 *Sciatic nerve*

29 *Hip/back/sciatic nerve*
30 *Ovary/testicle*
31 *Pelvic area*
32 *Lower back*
33 *Lymph/groin/Fallopian tube*
34 *Breast/lung*
35 *Arm/shoulder*
36 *Sinus/head/brain*
37 *Knee/leg/hip/lower back*
38 *Prostate/uterus/ rectum/sciatic nerve*
39 *Uterus/prostate*
40 *Sacrum/coccyx*
41 *Lumbar region*
42 *Thoracic region*
43 *Chest/lung/breast/back/ (on my left foot only) heart*

How does it work?

There is as yet no unified theory as to how reflexology works. But reflexologists believe that the benefits of the therapy are likely to derive from some or all of the following processes:

- deep muscle relaxation and the relief of tension and stress;
- an improvement in cardiovascular and lymphatic circulations;
- stimulation and inhibition of the transmission of nerve impulses to the brain, particularly those involving the autonomic nervous system;
- the reduction of pain through gate control (for details on the gate theory of pain, see page 79) and stimulation of the production of endorphins;
- stimulation of the key points on the acupuncture meridians;
- effects on the body's electromagnetic field;
- the benefits of an hour's rest and quiet;
- the psychological benefits of an hour's personal attention and care.

At home

You are likely to gain the most benefit from a reflexology massage, but you may achieve some relief by working some of the reflexology points yourself. Ask your practitioner to show you what to do, and to confirm that you can do this safely.

Walk barefoot as much as you can. Walking around the house will naturally massage and stimulate your reflexology points. Similarly if you walk barefoot outdoors on grass, sand, earth or smooth rocks, you will help to raise your body's energy levels and sense of wellbeing.

A modern, high-tech version of reflexology called Vacuflex uses a vacuum pump and suction to mimic the effect of the reflexologist's hands.

Biofeedback

The arthritis sufferer can benefit from biofeedback, where brain wave and other physiological activities are monitored to enable conscious control of normally unconscious functions.

The technique of biofeedback was first developed in the USA in 1958 by Joseph Kamiya, using existing electro-encephalogram (EEG) machines, which measure brain activity. Kamiya was researching the processes of sleep and dreaming and, because he was interested in the nature of human consciousness, he used an EEG to detect dreaming sleep. He found that the people in his study were able to alter their states of mind and achieve the alpha rate (the regular rhythm of brain waves in people at rest) by using his feedback from an adjacent room.

With biofeedback, people bring about their own physiological changes in conscious or unconscious ways. Nobody knows exactly how or why it works. It is believed that people use the feedback of information to change, and keep changing, what they do until they achieve the state or feeling they want (in the case of arthritis sufferers, the relief of pain). Physiological changes combined with the pleasure and sense of power derived from positive self-control are believed to be key factors in the success of biofeedback.

Today, purpose-built biofeedback instruments are extremely sophisticated. The visual or auditory response of a highly sensitive machine allows you to perceive unconscious – or involuntary – physiological (bodily) functions, which include heart rate, skin temperature and brain waves. The advantage of the procedure is that as soon as a machine is wired up, you receive instant, accurate feedback on your state of health. For example, you can see at once if your

heart or pulse is racing or if your body temperature has risen above normal.

An experienced biofeedback practitioner will teach you how to use the machine. Initially, the practitioner will teach you how to relax and slow down your functions so that stress and anxiety are reduced. Afterward, patients can purchase their own machines and use the skills they have learned at home in their everyday lives, thereby taking responsibility for their own health.

Biofeedback is typically used to alleviate specific medical conditions, as well as to help people cope with stress. It can also activate the relaxation response, so that the body's immune system can enhance and encourage the process of self-healing.

For arthritis sufferers, the main benefit is the control and relief of pain. Because your relaxation responses are accurately measured with the biofeedback technique, you can see for yourself how (or if) you are calming down. This enables you to control your own level of pain and may also help you to lessen your reliance on painkilling drugs.

Biofeedback machines do not alter brain waves or change muscle or heart activity. Using the machine is like stepping on to the bathroom scales to get an immediate record of your weight – the biofeedback machine gives you readings of your bodily functions.

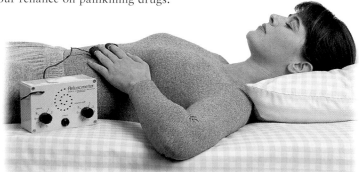

Dance therapy

The power of movement and dance has long been recognized as being of tremendous benefit to those who are not well, either physically or emotionally.

Arthritis sufferers can profit greatly by attending some form of dance class or dance exercise group. The enjoyment of music and rhythm is one of the world's great pleasures. Music seems to unlock the very energy in the human body, stimulating, motivating, supporting and balancing it. Dance helps to strengthen muscles and joints, and regulates the breathing and circulation. On a social level, it encourages partners to form relationships. In today's fast-paced life, it is sometimes easy to overlook the benefits of creative movement and dance.

Any form of dance therapy is a valuable treatment both for those with arthritis conditions and for those feeling under the weather, as many people with chronic arthritis often are.

The Medau movement

Heinrich Medau was a teacher of music and physical education who founded his own teacher-training college in Berlin in 1929. Medau was an enthusiastic and expert exponent of the new mode of rhythmic movement as a path to fitness, which was gradually replacing the old forms of rigid, army-style exercise.

Medau had taught and studied children's movement, observing that it was effortless, economical, elastic and "continuous through the body". He wished to preserve this natural talent into adulthood. As a music teacher Medau was aware of the individual's instinctive responses to – and enjoyment of – rhythm. He believed that "rhythm is the key to correct movement".

He developed a movement that was influenced by an enthusiasm for returning to nature, along with the less strict and rigid approach to education advocated by such teachers as Rudolf Steiner, who introduced the movement therapy eurythmy, Johann Pestalozzi and Maria Montessori. In the dance world, Isadora Duncan, with her free dance to natural rhythms, was another great influence.

The Medau movement is a formalized but natural system of dance, which has developed from the structure of the body itself rather than imposing upon it any distortion or rigidity. The techniques of this system are strong, rhythmical and dynamic, without jerky repetitions or overstretching. The main aim is to produce a lithe, strong body completely at ease and in harmony with itself. It has been adapted for work with the elderly as well as in physiotherapy and remedial classes, fitness courses and dance. It is also a valuable part of the repertoire of the healing therapies.

When you first attend a class, it is important that you tell your teacher the nature of your arthritis and how much you feel you are able to do. Do not be disheartened if you feel that this does not amount to very much at first. If you persist, you will find that you will be able to dance with greater mobility and suppleness as the weeks go by.

Other dance therapies

One of the newest complementary therapies to evolve this century is dance movement therapy, and this has been

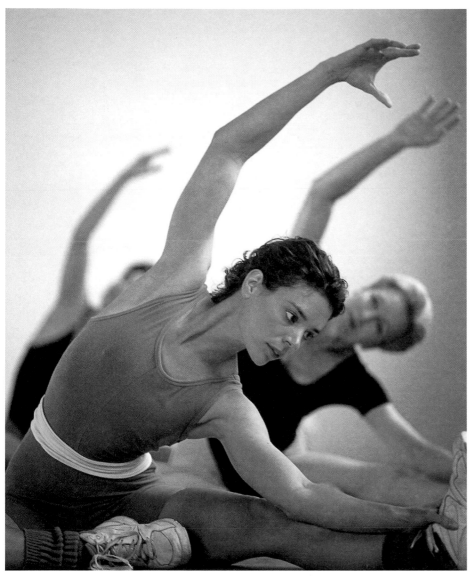

Dance therapy can be as formal or as informal as you want it to be. You don't have to be an expert to gain enjoyment and benefit from moving in time to music.

developed from the theories of Rudolph Laban. The therapy is designed to enable people to express their feelings, with a view to harmonizing both body and mind, through the power of movement.

It is unlikely that any one class will be the same as another, and this is one of the great joys of dance therapy. You are encouraged to express your individuality, your body's need to loosen up and regain mobility and your human need to respond to music. The need for physical contact is fulfilled in dance therapy to profound therapeutic effect.

Other types of dance may be equally suitable for people with arthritis. These include jazz dance and dancercise, to name just two that may be available at your local adult education centre. Ballroom dancing can be equally beneficial to arthritis sufferers – if you don't know how to do it, why not learn?

Colour therapy

According to colour therapists, colour affects not only our moods and feelings, but also our physical health and wellbeing. It is known that the colour scheme of a room can affect our moods, so perhaps it's not so surprising that colour may have some impact on our immune system – which can be affected by our emotions – and, therefore, our health.

The theory of colour therapy suggests that the body absorbs colour in the form of electromagnetic components of light, then produces its own aura of electromagnetism. This aura gives off a pattern of vibrations that can be discerned by a skilled colour therapist. A healthy body gives out a balanced pattern of vibrations, while an unhealthy body produces one that is unbalanced. The goal of the colour therapist is to administer the colour or colours that the sick person lacks in order to restore a balanced pattern to the aura.

The human aura is said to be ovoid in shape and made up of seven layers, the first of these being the physical body.

Colour therapists sometimes use a torch, in which light is shone through coloured, stained glass filters and directed on to specific chakras of the body.

Each of these layers interpenetrates others and is filled with ever-changing colours. These changes depend on our state of health and our moods. When we become angry, for example, our aura turns a murky red, and when we are envious it takes on a dark shade of green.

Disease first manifests itself in the aura, and it can be seen as a grey mass of accumulated energy. If this is not resolved, it will continue to manifest itself and become a physical symptom in the body. Once it reaches this stage, the colour therapist will have to disperse this mass of stagnant energy by reintroducing the colour frequency into both the physical body and the aura.

Colour therapists tend to regard their therapy as complementary to orthodox medical treatment but some have a measure of success in treating arthritis. The colours most frequently used are red, orange, gold, yellow, green, turquoise, blue, indigo, violet and magenta. Colour treatment can be administered either through a colour therapy instrument, which uses stained glass for filters, or through contact healing. In contact healing, the therapist allows his or her body to be the instrument through which colour is channelled to the patient.

Prana

The traditional therapies practised in India and Sri Lanka are based on the ideal of *prana*, literally breath, but meaning vital energy. *Prana* is equivalent to *qi* in Chinese and *ki* in Japanese. The most important function within the human body is the transference of prana, or life energy. Prana is absorbed into the body in many ways, including through the breath and through the food we eat.

Prana vitalizes the etheric layer of the aura that surrounds and interpenetrates with the physical body. The etheric is the blueprint for the physical body and contains the major and minor chakras and the nadis. The word *chakra* is Sanskrit for "wheel or vortex of energy". *Nadis* are energetic pathways that link the chakras through the body.

Five of the major chakras are situated in line with the spine, the sixth with the brow and the seventh lies just above the crown of the head. Prana is absorbed through the splenic chakra. On entering this centre, it is refracted into the colours of the spectrum, which are then transferred to the appropriate major chakra. Each of the major chakras contains the full spectrum of colour, with one colour being dominant in each. Apart from being associated with various parts of the physical body, each chakra is linked to one of the endocrine glands, and this is the reason for their importance in treatment. The nadis are linked with our nervous system and are the fine energy channels through which prana flows.

On a sunny day there is an abundance of prana in the atmosphere, which is one of the reasons why we feel so full of energy on those days. On a grey dull winter's day, prana is greatly reduced.

The consultation

The colour therapist will take a detailed medical and life history from you and ask you about your arthritis condition, your lifestyle, your diet and how you exercise.

The first part of the treatment involves making a colour-diagnosis spine chart (see box below). The therapist may also work with crystals of different colours and coloured water.

The colour therapist will feel and work with your aura to disperse any energy blockages and then lay hands over your body to allow the appropriate colours to be channelled into it.

At home

Once you know which colours are best for you, you can continue the treatment at home by wearing clothes of that colour or by wearing a piece of silk or cotton of the appropriate colour. Natural fibres are used because synthetic fabrics restrict the aura. You can also incorporate favourable colours into your home decor. Gemstones may be used in colour therapy as well.

Find out more

Yoga	*44–47*
Choosing a	
practitioner	*106–107*

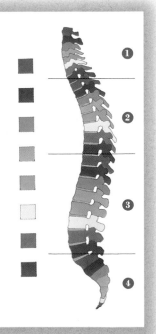

COLOUR DIAGNOSTIC CHART

The spine is divided into four sections, each containing eight vertebrae. Each section relates to aspects of your health: the first section to mental health; the second, to emotional health; the third, to your metabolism; and the fourth, to physical health. Each vertebra within a section is assigned one of the colours of the spectrum. The chart is used to determine the overall colour needed plus information on your general condition.

Counselling and psychotherapy

The benefits of counselling are widely accepted – in fact, counselling is now automatically offered to ayone who has experienced a traumatic event or who is facing incurable illness.

Complementary therapists recognize that successful healing depends on treating the mind as much as it does the body. Having someone you trust, such as a best friend, to whom you can talk about your troubles is a first step towards feeling better.

Counselling and psychotherapy are not so much alternative answers to treating arthritis as they are complementary supports. Indeed, many – if not all – conventional family doctors and hospital consultants would acknowledge the power of the mind over the body and would approve if you decide to seek some form of counselling to help you cope with a severe, chronic illness.

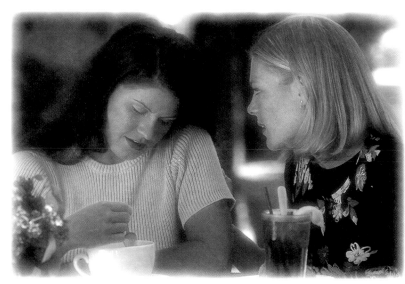

The mind–body link

It is now well established that there is a powerful link between the workings of the mind and the body. A new science called psychoneuroimmunology has proved that the immune system and other parts of the body respond to negative and positive thoughts and thinking styles. Research shows that the immune system is adversely affected by stress, particularly by major crises such as bereavement or divorce, and that stress produces chemical changes within the body. These changes are scientifically measurable. It has also been shown that psychotherapeutic techniques can strengthen the immune system and help ward off disease.

The therapies described here all subscribe to the concept of the mind affecting the body. Some therapists maintain that everyone has the potential to achieve total good health, with freedom from disease. However, an unhealthy lifestyle, a gloomy environment and negative emotions and thinking styles can all contribute to disease.

This theory works in reverse, too. Once arthritis is established, it can affect your mood and emotions. Constant pain is tiring and stressful. Long-term stress can produce depression and other psychological states, which could be alleviated with professional help.

Pain clinics and programmes for the relief of chronic pain include a psychological component because your emotional wellbeing has a significant effect on both how you see your pain and how you cope with it. Psychotherapy is essentially a "talking cure" and can be divided into three types:
• supportive psychotherapy
• exploratory psychotherapy
• specialized psychotherapy.

Supportive psychotherapy

This is the simplest and least intrusive of the psychotherapies. The client simply talks about his or her problems in an atmosphere of trust and confidentiality. This is a vital ingredient in complementary therapies and in medical consultations, whether the illness is acute or chronic, curable or incurable.

Exploratory psychotherapy

Here the client is encouraged to explore the problem rather than merely voice it. The therapist will actively intervene to point out inconsistencies, evasions and neglected aspects of an issue. If this is done diplomatically – without losing the warmth and lack of bias that are the hallmarks of supportive psychotherapy – exploratory psychotherapy can be a powerful, positive instrument for changing your perceptions and methods for coping with pain from arthritis.

Before you begin exploratory psychotherapy, a structure should be established. You should discuss with your therapist the goals that you expect to achieve, and the number and length of the sessions necessary for you to reach them.

Specialist psychotherapies

Behavioural psychotherapy, cognitive therapy, psychoanalysis, gestalt, psychodrama (drama therapy) and many less well-known therapies are all specialist psychotherapies. The psychotherapy that is most suitable for people with arthritis is cognitive therapy, which can challenge negative habits and thought, solve problems and help people think more positively. It is one of the most powerful tools for fighting chronic pain and for coping with disability and immobility.

Cognitive therapy was introduced by American psychiatrist Aaron Beck nearly 30 years ago. Its aim is to use positive thinking to alter a person's perceptions, memories and thoughts about themselves in order to help them cope more successfully with their lives.

Positive thinking, in essence, means focusing on the good things in your life and paying as little attention as possible to the bad things. This is the basis of the affirmations technique used in various psychological therapies. It does not matter what the affirmation is, provided that it is positive in outlook. Positive thinking is specifically designed to raise your self-esteem and, consequently, your general state of health.

The psychotherapist will suggest you remind yourself each morning:
• I am alive and capable of enjoying life.
• I enjoy doing ... (you choose what the affirmation is to be).
• I enjoy seeing ... (you choose which of your friends and family it is to be).
• I enjoy looking at ... (pictures, films, television programmes – you choose).
• Today I am looking forward to ... (you decide).

Make up your own list of the positive things in your life and repeat them to yourself every morning and whenever you have an attack of pain. Try not to focus on the pain. Concentrate on the positive.

How to find a psychotherapist

You can find a therapist by asking your family doctor or hospital consultant, or you can obtain a recommendation from a friend. Whoever you decide to see, check their credentials with a governing body.

Find out more
Managing the pain   *138–141*
Choosing a
*   practitioner*   *106–107*

OTHER PSYCHOLOGICAL THERAPIES

If you believe that the mind plays a powerful part in healing the body, you could also consider:
• *Aromatherapy (see page 50)*
• *Meditation (see page 54)*
• *Visualization (see page 56)*
• *Relaxation (see page 58)*
• *Self-hypnosis (see page 60)*
• *Biofeedback (see page 99)*

Choosing a practitioner

*F*inding the right complementary practitioner is an important step. It is worthwhile to do extensive homework to ensure you find a good therapist, and to establish at the beginning whether a rapport will develop between the two of you.

It is worth making extensive enquiries about any therapist before committing yourself to what could be an expensive course of treatment.

Conventional doctors and dentists must be registered with their professional councils; in turn, these councils, are responsible for inspecting colleges and setting standards and professional discipline. Although osteopaths and chiropractors are regulated, this is not always true for other therapies. It is important, especially when suffering from a chronic or severe condition such as arthritis, that you check your therapist's qualifications, training and experience with a governing body. Certificates on the wall may mean little in practice, so follow your intuition. If you don't feel comfortable with a therapist's credentials, look for another one elsewhere.

Many health centres and hospitals have complementary practitioners attached to them. Before going to an unknown therapist, ask your doctor what is available through the surgery. Some health professionals practise complementary therapies themselves – general practitioners may prescribe homeopathy, nurses may use aromatherapy and physiotherapists may perform acupuncture.

Your therapist should be knowledgeable about the nature of arthritis. It sometimes helps if the therapist has had

personal experience of the condition. In fact, many complementary therapists train in a particular discipline after they themselves have been helped by it. This tends to give the treatment they are offering more credibility.

Meeting the therapist

The treatments given by a complementary therapist can work in subtle ways, so it is important that you and your therapist can work together in harmony and that your practitioner has some empathy with your condition. Some research suggests that the therapist can be just as important as the therapy itself. If you do not feel an instant rapport with your therapist, it is best to seek help from someone else.

Before signing up for an expensive and protracted course of treatment, check whether your therapist is happy to work with your conventional doctor and whether the treatments are covered under any health insurance schemes. Many are these days, especially if you have been referred by your doctor. Therapies such as acupuncture, osteopathy, homeopathy and the Alexander technique have become accepted by conventional doctors and are available under a number of schemes. You should insist on knowing in advance how many treatments you are likely to need, and how much this is likely to cost. Ask precisely how the treatment offered is likely to benefit your arthritis.

The therapist's premises do not have to be luxurious – perhaps you should be on your guard if they are, as that could mean they are making too much money out of their clients – but they should be clean and tidy. If you are not satisfied with what you find, don't book any sessions. Always be wary of any hard-sell methods, or attempts to make you buy expensive extras, such as dietary supplements, books and videos.

Once you have begun a course of treatment, the therapist should keep to the times of your appointments, and be as efficient and practical as any other doctor. Although you cannot expect to feel better immediately, you should be able to observe progress as you continue with the treatments.

The great majority of complementary practitioners are honest, decent people who want to help restore your health. They are also understandably enthusiastic about the treatments they can offer. However, arthritis is currently incurable and may always return. There are no miracle cures, so never book sessions with any practitioner who claims to be able to get rid of your arthritis for ever.

Find out more

Choosing a complementary
  therapy   *42–43*
Helpful organizations   *155*

QUESTIONS YOU SHOULD ASK

When deciding on a new practitioner, contact the relevant school, college and/or professional organization to find out everything you can about his or her qualifications. Some therapies have more than one professional body, and one may have less strict requirements than another. If you are in any doubt, look elsewhere for treatment. When you first contact a new practitioner, ask the following questions before making a decision to see him or her for treatment:

* *What qualifications do you have, and when and where did you obtain them?*

* *Do you belong to a professional body? (If he or she doesn't, be very wary.)*

* *If there is no professional body for your field, how are you and others in your profession regulated? (Is your practitioner on any form of register, for example, or does he or she practise through a respectable clinic?)*

* *How long have you been practising? Have you kept up to date with advances in knowledge since you have qualified?*

* *What do you know about my form of arthritis?*

* *Have you already had successes in treating people with any form of arthritis? Can I speak to any of these people?*

* *Do you think you can bring about a significant improvement in my condition? If so, how long is treatment likely to take, and what will it cost?*

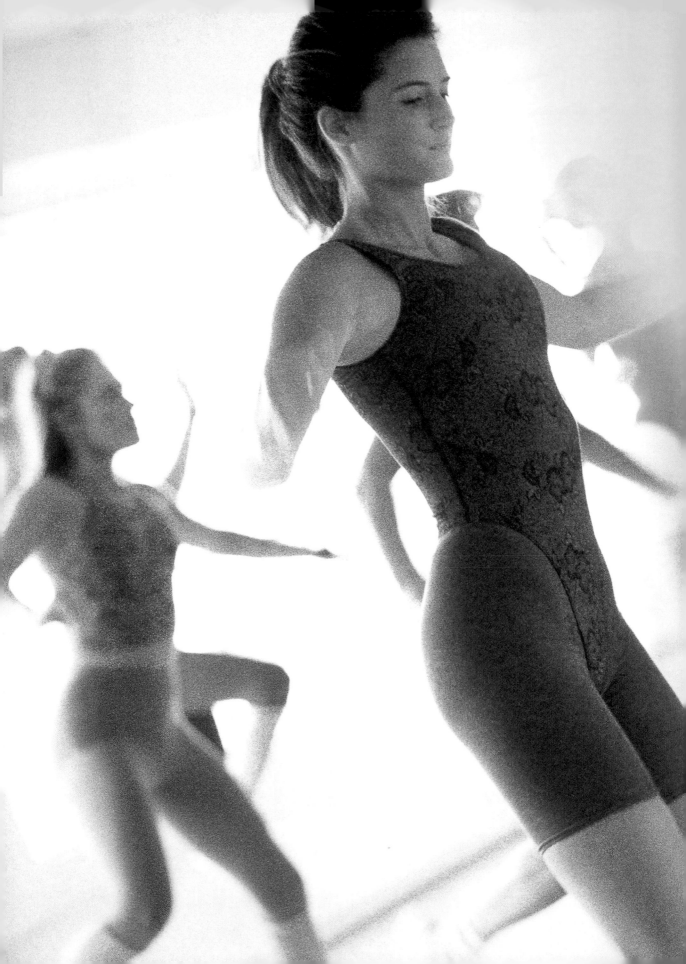

3

CONVENTIONAL

TREATMENTS

It must be said that arthritis is not curable. However, with the many different choices available, there is no reason for you to suffer from pain. Among the conventional treatments for arthritis are: medication, losing weight, exercise, electrical therapies (such as TENS), occupational therapy and the surgical options. No doubt other treatments will become available within the next few years.

For some people, surgery is really and truly the only choice. However, the joy of being transformed from being immobile to being able to walk around unaided, through the means of a hip replacement, for example, can hardly be overestimated.

Drug therapy

Despite the undeniable growth in popularity of alternative remedies, it is with drugs that arthritis is most commonly treated. For anyone taking drugs to control an arthritic condition, understanding the differences between the various types of drugs and the effects that they may have is vital.

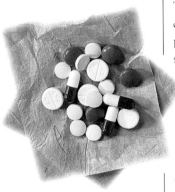

The range of painkillers on the market is wide and can be confusing, and you may need to take a combination of drugs. Make sure you only take ones recommended by your doctor. Taking the wrong drugs can make matters worse rather than better.

There are a vast array of drugs that you can buy over the counter or that may be prescribed to combat the pain and symptoms of an arthritic condition. These can be roughly divided into three categories: those which reduce the pain, those which reduce inflammation and pain, and those which reduce disease activity and tackle inflammation. To treat your particular problem, you may have take a combination of drugs or undergo trial periods to ascertain the effectiveness of the treatments. Always pay special attention to any side effects associated with a drug.

Painkillers

Analgesics, or painkillers, relieve pain by interfering with the messages being transmitted to the brain via the network of nerve fibres in the body. There are two main groups of painkillers: simple analgesics, such as aspirin, and narcotic analgesics, including codeine and morphine. Most painkillers you buy over the counter are of the non-narcotic type. Some, such as ibuprofen, are actually non-steroidal anti-inflammatory (NSAIDs). Many brand-name painkillers are made by combining aspirin with other non-narcotic drugs, such as caffeine, or with mild narcotic drugs such as codeine to produce "compound painkillers".

Be careful about mixing analgesics: by taking two different brands of painkillers you may exceed the recommended dose for one of the ingredients. It is best to avoid alcohol when taking analgesics, and long-term use of these drugs should be medically supervised. Because analgesics mask pain, it is also important to avoid overusing a joint when taking them.

INFLAMMATORY ARTHRITIS – VITAL EARLY TREATMENT

Not long ago there was some debate as to whether early, aggressive therapy made any difference to the outcome of patients with inflammatory arthritis, including rheumatoid arthritis. Treatment tended to be based on the idea of first- and second-line drugs, beginning with NSAIDs and progressing to DMARDs such as gold, suphasalazine and methrotrexate. Most rheumatologists are now convinced that accurate diagnosis and appropriate intervention with drugs and physiotherapy in the early stage of the disease are crucial, because the longer inflammation lasts, the more damage is caused. This means patients are now more likely to be prescribed one or more disease-modifying drugs early on. Doctors argue that once inflammation is suppressed, patients will not deteriorate and should actually improve. Patients also seem less likely to suffer side-effects from these drugs if they are treated sooner rather than later.

NSAIDs

Non-steroidal anti-inflammatory drugs (NSAIDs) reduce inflammation as well as pain. Their main role in the treatment of arthritis is to reduce inflammation in the joint linings, thereby reducing swelling and relieving pain and stiffness. If no inflammation is present, as is often the case in osteoarthritis, NSAIDs may have no advantage over analgesics. That said, they are used for many different types of arthritis, often with other drugs. This is because they provide relief from symptoms, although they do not modify the course of the disease. NSAIDs can have some side effects, and you may have to take them with food or milk.

DMARDs

Disease-modifying anti-rheumatic drugs (DMARDs) play a key role in the treatment of rheumatoid arthritis. They may also be used in some other types of rheumatic diseases, such as ankylosing spondylitis or the arthritis linked with psoriasis. DMARDs lower disease activity and inflammation, thereby reducing pain, swelling and stiffness of joints, and they are often effective in cases where anti-inflammatory drugs are not. However, they have potentially more damaging side-effects than NSAIDs.

DMARDs tend to be slow-acting and it may take weeks or even months for the full benefit to be felt. As they are not analgesics you may have to carry on with painkillers or with anti-inflammatory drugs.

Steroids

Corticosteroids, often shortened to steroids, are hormones; some are produced naturally in the body, others manufactured synthetically. Those used in the treatment of arthritis are derived from, or are synthetic variants of, the natural corticosteroid hormones formed in the outer part of the adrenal glands.

When present in large amounts, corticosteroids reduce inflammation and suppress immune responses – which is why they are used for patients with rheumatoid arthritis and other types of rheumatic disease.

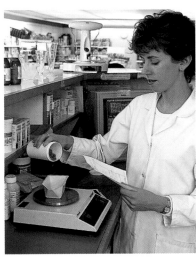

Always tell your doctor and pharmacist about any medicines you are currently taking – both prescribed and over the counter. They will be able to offer invaluable advice on which drugs are the most appropriate for your particular circumstances.

OSTEOARTHRITIS AND GENE THERAPY

People used to think osteoarthritis was an inevitable part of ageing, due to wear and tear. However, research funded by the Arthritis Research Campaign (ARC) in the United Kingdom has shown there is a definite disease process – which means that if there is a cause, there may be a cure. Paul Dieppe, professor of rheumatology at Bristol University, describes osteoarthritis as "joint failure". As in the case of heart failure, there may be many different factors that develop together to cause joints to break down – these include gait, weight, injury and patterns of work. The question remained, why did some people exposed to the these factors suffer and not others? ARC-funded research at Thomas's Hospital, London, has shown that genetic factors also play a vital part. Now researchers are working to find the gene or genes responsible so that new methods of early diagnosis and treatment can be developed.

Drug therapy

DRUGS USED TO TREAT PAIN

DRUG TYPE	NAME	EFFECTS AND SIDE-EFFECTS
SIMPLE ANALGESICS	Aspirin	Relieves pain in body tissues, such as muscles, ligaments and joints, particularly when associated with inflammation. Can be taken in pill form or, most effectively, dissolved in water. May irritate the stomach and, if taken on a long-term basis, may cause stomach ulcers.
	Paracetamol	An effective painkiller, but does not relieve inflammation. Is preferred treatment for osteoarthritis because it has fewer side-effects than aspirin or NSAIDs. Overdosing can result in serious liver and kidney damage.
COMPOUND PAINKILLERS	Benoral	A compound of aspirin and paracetamol which delivers a regular quantity of both drugs into the bloodstream. An effective painkiller which also relieves inflammation, it is very useful in the treatment of arthritis. For side effects, see aspirin and paracetamol above.
NARCOTIC ANALGESICS	Morphine Dihydrocodeine Co-proxamol (Distalgesic) Diamorphine	Not routinely used for people with long-term rheumatic disorders, but may be prescribed to relieve moderate or severe pain. Side-effects can include nausea, vomiting, drowsiness, constipation and, occasionally, breathing difficulties. Some are very powerful and long-term use can lead to tolerance and dependence.

DRUGS USED TO TREAT PAIN

DRUG TYPE	NAME	EFFECTS AND SIDE-EFFECTS
NSAIDs (non-steroidal anti-inflammatory drugs)	indomethacin (Indocid) naproxen (Naprosyn) ibuprofen (Brufen/Nurofen) fenbufen (Lederfen) piroxicam (Feldene) diclofenac (Voltarol)	Reduce inflammation in the joint linings, thereby reducing swelling and relieving pain and stiffness. If no inflammation is present, as is often the case in osteoarthritis, NSAIDs may have no advantage over analgesics. They are often used for arthritis with other drugs as they provide relief from symptoms, although they do not modify the course of the disease. NSAIDS are usually taken by mouth as tablets or capsules, although many are available as a liquid suspension or suppository. A slow release or "retard" preparation often helps to relieve early-morning joint stiffness. Some also come in the form of rub-in gels. Side effects include the risk of developing gastro-intestinal problems such as ulcers, nausea, stomach and bowel upsets, heartburn and indigestion, or allergic reactions such as rashes and wheeziness, fluid retention and, rarely, kidney damage or blood disorders. To minimize any side effects, take NSAIDs with or after food, and with a glass of fluid. Keep your alchol and caffeine intake to a minimum and do not smoke.
	meloxicam (Mobic)	This is a newer type of NSAID, more narrowly targeted on inflamed tissues, which has a lesser effect on the stomach and intestine. It may be a sensible choice for those who have stomach problems relating to NSAID use.

Drug therapy

DRUGS USED TO TREAT PAIN

DRUG TYPE	NAME	EFFECTS AND SIDE EFFECTS
STEROIDS	Hydrocortisone Prednisolone Triamcinolone Methylprednisolone	-Steroids are manufactured versions of hormones produced naturally in the adrenal glands. Corticosteroids reduce inflammation and suppress immune responses. Steroids can be given in tablet form or by injection into an inflamed joint, and can help with sudden flare-ups. Side effects from injections can include a flare-up in joint pain within the first 24 hours after the injection, infection in the joint following injection and thinning of the skin at the injection site with peri-articular injections. Side effects from oral steriods include bloating, cramps, weight gain, a round "moon" face, stretch marks or thinning of the skin, cataracts, blood pressure and sleep problems and osteoporosis. Because the body becomes dependent on oral steroids, they should only be reduced gradually.

DRUGS USED TO TREAT PAIN

DRUG TYPE	NAME	EFFECTS AND SIDE EFFECTS
DMARDs (disease modifying antirheumatic drugs), also known as disease controlling antirheumatic therapy (DCART)		DMARDs suppress the disease process and ease symptoms such as inflammation.
	Nethotrexate	An immunosuppressant, originally used to treat cancer, nethotrexate is an effective and increasingly used drug for rheumatoid arthritis. It is usually taken by mouth, but also by injection. Side effects include nausea and diarrhoea, blood disorders and liver damage. As with most DMARDS, have regular check-ups, especially when starting this drug.
	Sulphasalazine	Combination of an antibiotic and aspirin used to suppress rheumatic inflammation, sulphasalazine may cause rashes, gastro-intestinal and blood disorders and may stain contact lenses.
	Gold sodium aurothiomalate (Myocrisin) Auranofin	Gold can be given in the form of injections or by mouth. Injections will be given as an initial test dose, then weekly thereafter. Taking gold orally tends to be less effective and can take some months to become effective. Side effects include blood, kidney and skin disorders, rash, mouth ulcers, sore throat, fever, bruising, breathlessness and diarrhoea.
	Penicillamine	Taken orally, at least an hour before food. Can alter your sense of taste, but this should diminish after a few weeks. Otherwise side effects are as above.
	Antimalarials hydroxychloroquine chloroquine	Effective for rheumatoid arthritis and systemic lupus erythematosus. Side effects are uncommon, the most serious concern being damage to the retina.

Physical therapies

There are many ways in which you can take control of some of the factors that may be affecting your arthritis. Losing weight can have profound implications on the severity of your symptoms.

Humans are designed to be slim rather than flabby and the Western epidemic of obesity is causing an increase in many disease conditions, including arthritis.

Following a sensible diet to lose weight can be reinforced by keeping a diary of everything that you eat. Once you have reached a healthy weight, maintain your routine to keep it off.

Being overweight is a proven risk factor in arthritis. Any suspension system wears out more quickly if it is overburdened. Being overweight can put unnatural strains on joints. Tendons and ligaments may become separated by layers of fat, distorting the ways in which they connect with the bones. Fat people are usually less active than thin people, and this, too, has a bad effect in arthritis. Moderate, regular exercise helps in arthritis.

Keeping your weight under control has several advantages for arthritis sufferers. It lessens the burden on load-bearing joints, especially the hips and knees and between the vertebrae of the spine. It may make you feel younger. Keeping your weight under control can give a big psychological boost to people with arthritis, as well as improving their general health.

Are you overweight?

One way to find out if you are overweight by visiting your family doctor or hospital outpatient's department, where there will usually be a weighing machine with clearly marked indications of what is mildly and seriously overweight for someone of your height and gender. You will be advised on how much to lose and over

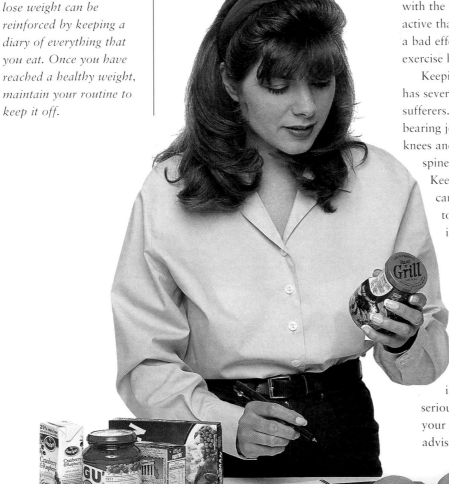

what period of time according to what your weight is. Another way is to find your body mass index (see box, below).

If you are within a healthy weight limit, do not try to lose weight to combat or avoid arthritis. You may do yourself more harm than good.

How much weight to lose

It is important not to try to lose a lot of weight in a short time. Research shows, conclusively, that rapid weight loss is almost invariably followed by rapid weight gain, sometimes to a greater weight than the weight that the person was originally. Crash or severely restricted diets are, therefore, unhelpful. You should follow a sensible diet, ideally recommended or approved by your doctor or specialist nurse.

Someone who is very overweight may initially lose weight rapidly, but once that first phase is completed after a month or so, the best long-term rate of loss is 0.5 to 1.0 kilograms (1 to 2 pounds) each week. Younger and taller people will usually find the upper limit achievable. Older,

shorter people may have to be content with a rate of loss near the bottom limit. You may like to keep a chart, which acts both as a motivator and a reminder, to record your weight loss or decreasing BMI weekly. Support groups may be helpful.

Weight control requires discipline. Once the target has been reached, diet still has to be controlled. Partners, family and friends can help with encouraging comments. Most people like their appearance to be appreciated, and also like their determination and effort in keeping to the diet to be observed.

Fasting

Some complementary therapists recommend fasting as a treatment for arthritis in order to detoxify the system and eliminate long-accumulated waste products. Fasting should last no longer than three days unless you are under medical supervision. It is essential to drink a glass of water every hour when you are fasting. Fasting has no proven benefits for the treatment of arthritis.

BODY MASS INDEX

BMI, or body mass index, is a way of expressing someone's weight in relation to their height. It is now superseding the conventional height/weight tables, as it is believed to be a more reliable indication of desirable weight. It is obtained by dividing a person's weight in kilograms by the square of their height in metres. For example, this is the equation if you weigh 60 kg and are 1.6 m tall: 1.6 × 1.6 = 2.6; then 60 ÷ 2.6 = 23.1. (To convert from imperial measurements, multiply pounds by 0.45 to get kilograms and feet by 0.3 to get metres.)

A healthy weight is one in which the body mass index (BMI) is no more than 25. When the product of this reaches 25 the person involved is roughly at the top of what an insurance company calls their desirable weight range. A body mass index of between 18 and 25 indicates no discernible relationship between fatness and mortality. Above 25, however, the mortality ratio increases steadily until at 35 the risk of death is double that of people with a body mass index of 25.

Physiotherapy and exercise

Physiotherapy is widely used to treat stiff joints, a main symptom in some forms of arthritis. Carefully used with professional advice, it can be of considerable benefit to those suffering from rheumatoid arthritis and osteoarthritis.

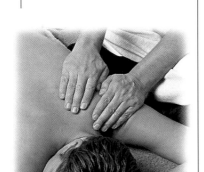

The pain associated with some types of arthritis can be relieved by a qualified physiotherapist. Care must be taken to ensure that the treatment is appropriate for the problem and not given excessively.

Muscles weakened as a consequence of inactivity through arthritis will benefit from physiotherapy. The techniques used can include passive exercise, in which the therapist moves the affected part of a joint to preserve joint mobility, or active exercise, in which the arthritis sufferer is taught to exercise those muscles that are most in need of exercise. You can do this for yourself to a modest degree; to get your joints going in the morning, when they tend to be the most stiff, take a warm bath and do some moderate exercise.

Physiotherapy can help to treat stretched ligaments, maintain smooth joint functioning and prevent deformities developing. Manipulation can also be valuable. Therapeutic massage – from a qualified person – can also help to treat the symptoms of arthritis, particularly muscular pain (see pages 68–73).

Physiotherapy is frequently prescribed for lower back pain in arthritis sufferers. Where it is not appropriate, the emphasis is on rest, support and controlled "ordinary" exercise.

People with an extremely severe arthritis disability may benefit from physiotherapy, but they may still suffer from restricted mobility. For these people, there is a range of physical aids available that can help them cope with everyday activities (see pages 152–153). Hydrotherapy – exercise in water – is also beneficial.

Taking exercise

It is worth remembering that someone with arthritis needs exercise for the same reasons as everyone else: to maintain muscle power and tone, and the range of movement around the joints, to keep a happy balance between mental and physical activity, to keep the heart in healthy condition and to raise the level of endorphins (the body's natural painkillers) in order to minimize pain and keep you feeling cheerful.

For rheumatoid arthritis sufferers, exercise can be a mixed blessing. On the one hand, rest reduces inflammation, on the other hand, rest over long periods allows muscles to weaken, joints to become stiff and bones to weaken. The solution is to take some exercise, but to do so carefully and only as long as it doesn't hurt too much.

Osteoarthritis is usually much more constant in its symptoms than rheumatoid arthritis. It is without doubt linked to body weight, and weight control is an important factor in the management of the condition (see pages 116–117). This should be undertaken in conjunction with regular exercise. However, joint damage which is caused partly by stress on the joints should not be compounded by over-strenuous exercise.

You will find your own levels of exercise – what you can and cannot do – through your own common sense and experience. You should undertake activities that improve the general tone of muscles, rather than those designed to increase muscular strength; for example, walking, swimming and gardening, such as pruning and watering plants, are more suitable than press-ups, weightlifting or digging in heavy soils.

It is important to make the mental and physical effort needed to keep taking moderate exercise, even if this involves some moderate level of pain. Exercise should be regular and, if possible, gradually progressive, provided that it does not lead to severe pain. Aim for three or four sessions of 20–30 minutes each week. Self-discipline – for example, setting aside the same time every day to take exercise – ensures that you get regular exercise to prevent joints becoming harmfully stiff.

Anyone affected by rheumatic finger joints knows that they need exercising regularly, that this usually involves some effort of will and that there may be times when the fingers can be moved almost freely and other times when they can hardly be moved at all. The best advice is that joints affected by any form of arthritis should be stretched to the limit of moderate discomfort several times each day, in order to avoid permanent stiffness developing. Effort without fanaticism is the key.

If a joint is splinted to relieve symptoms by preventing movement, it may be possible to use the splint only at night. This will allow moderate, controlled exercise during the day and help prevent further muscle wastage.

Find out more

Many health-care professionals believe that walking for 30 minutes every day is the best form of exercise. Walking with someone whose company you enjoy will encourage you to do it regularly, and make it a pleasant experience rather than a chore.

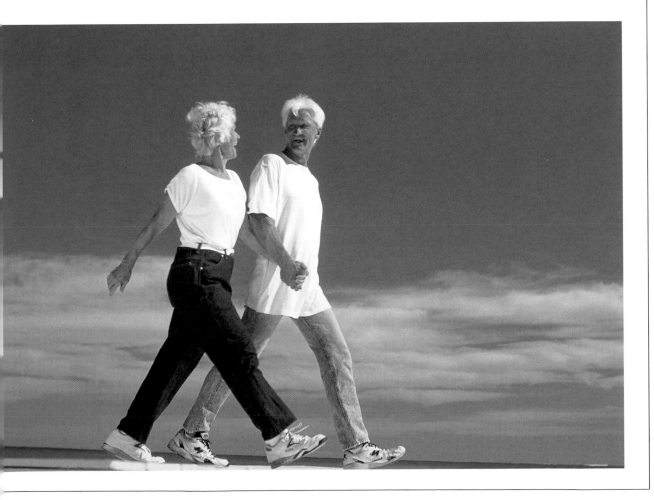

Electrical therapies

There are two main types of therapy that can be used to stimulate tissue in an area affected by arthritis. These are transcutaneous electrical nerve stimulation (TENS or TNS) and ultrasonic therapy.

Pain signals normally travel from the site of the stimulus via a peripheral nerve to the spinal cord then to the brain. One theory of how TENS works proposes that it makes specific cells in the spinal cord less responsive to pain signals, reducing the perception of pain in the brain. A second theory ascribes the pain-relieving effect to electrical impulses stimulating the release of endorphins, the brain's natural painkillers, which block the pain.

Transcutaneous electrical nerve stimulation, or TENS as it is commonly called, is used worldwide for the relief of chronic pain, including some forms of arthritis, as part of a total strategy for chronic pain control. It works by electrically stimulating nerve fibres in the skin, which helps to block or suppress pain messages to the brain.

TENS units, which are usually battery powered, are the size of small portable stereos and have controls for the frequency and amplitude of the current used. The current is passed into the skin via reusable rubber or self-adhesive electrodes. Some units have large rotary control knobs designed for people with arthritis of the hand.

The electrodes are placed on the skin in the affected area and a low-voltage current is passed through them, at first at a low level; the amplitude is then gradually increased and the frequency of the current is varied until it becomes just noticeably painful. The level is then adjusted to just below that point. The physiotherapist giving the treatment may test different frequencies to see which is most effective in relieving pain. Each treatment may vary from 20 minutes to 2 hours, and patients may require between three and five sessions before their pain is reduced.

About 60 per cent of people who try the treatment find it helpful in relieving pain. Some find that the relief is short-lived, but others find themselves relieved of pain for periods varying from several hours to several days, or weeks.

People who benefit from TENS may wish to buy their own equipment for use at home. TENS should be used only after checking with your doctor to make sure it is safe for you. It should not be used in the early stages of pregnancy or by someone fitted with a pacemaker.

Ultrasonic therapy

Effectively a form of massage, ultrasonic therapy for pain depends upon sound waves that are impelled into human tissue where they cause rapid, gentle vibration and slight local heating. As such waves travel through human tissue, different frequencies are absorbed by different tissues in the human body; for example, skin, fat, muscle and bone. One reason

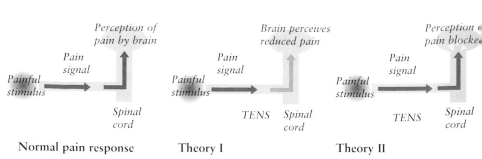

Normal pain response　　　**Theory I**　　　**Theory II**

for a frequency being well absorbed by a particular tissue is that it is the frequency at which the molecules of that tissue naturally vibrate.

Ultrasonic massage devices operate at frequencies designed to resonate with (that is, to set off sympathetic vibrations in) a wide range of human tissues. As sound waves travel through human tissues, their vibrations cause alternate loosening and tightening of cell walls. This stimulates the metabolism, and it can also improve blood circulation. Sound waves can have therapeutic effects on tissues beneath the surface of the body, including some that may be affected by arthritis, which may be difficult to treat with other therapies.

Find out more

Massage	*68–73*
Drug therapy	*110–115*
Managing the pain	*136–139*

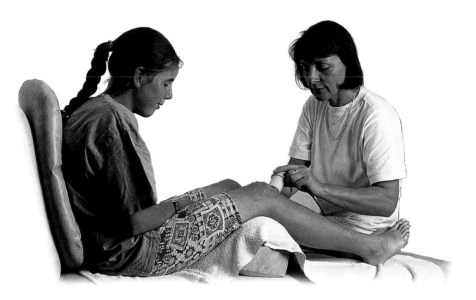

Stiffened joints can be relaxed through ultrasonic therapy. People with knee pain and lower back pain testify to benefits from this form of treatment.

CASE HISTORY

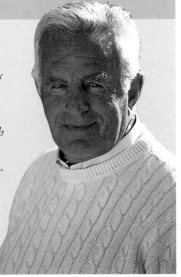

George, *who is 60 years of age, had had stiff, painful knees for years, which made standing up, sitting down and walking difficult. He also had a chronically painful stiff shoulder, and this made it difficult to reach up, for example, to remove items from high shelves and to change light bulbs.*

"My condition was not severe enough for surgery, but my life was painfully limited by my condition and, while I found painkilling and anti-inflammatory drugs useful, they did have side-effects, such as constipation, which could be a problem.

I decided it was worth seeking relief by using other forms of therapy. A physiotherapist suggested that I try transcutaneous nerve stimulation, which might help with my shoulder pain, and he referred me for a number of sessions. After a few of these the pain was reduced and my shoulder movement eased. I also used ultrasonic therapy to treat my knees and experienced relief from pain and stiffness."

Occupational therapy

Continuing to live a normal life and maintaining your personal independence while coping with arthritis is vital for your self-confidence and self-esteem. Visiting an occupational therapist will allow you to continue doing all you did before, but with some fundamental modifications. Take advantage of the advice that is on offer and shape a lifestyle which is appropriate to you.

If you visit a hospital for arthritis treatment, or go to a clinic, use part of your time there to discover how best to cope with any disability you may have and adapt this knowledge to your life at home. This will allow you to maintain your normal, everyday occupations as far as possible. You can derive much satisfaction and a sense of being in charge of your own life from adapting your home environment.

In addition to taking advice from your hospital's physiotherapist, ask your family doctor for referral to an occupational therapist. Occupational therapists will be able to recommend ways of doing things and gadgets that can help. Some ideas are described in this section and a therapist will recommend those that are particularly useful in your case.

Your therapist will be able to give you valuable advice on your own particular problems. He or she will help you with exercise problems and recurrent pain problems. You may be advised to use devices to avoid injury to weak joints. These may include wearing built-up shoes or wrist supports. The therapist will also help you with any problems associated with managing your life at home. This may be in the form of reorganizing your furniture; how you store common objects that you use every day; or gadgets to make certain tasks easier.

Getting dressed

Your problems are likely to start with getting up in the morning. The clothes you choose can help enormously, with the emphasis being on things that are easy to slip on or off, so as to avoid difficult, fiddly finger movements and having to bend down to the level of your feet. For example, a loose crew-neck jumper will be easier to pull over your head than a tight turtleneck jumper.

Slip-on shoes, zips with large, easy-to-hold pulls rather than buttons, Velcro fastenings and belts that hook rather than buckle all make life easier. You may have to invest in gadgets such as a long-handled shoehorn and a buttonhook to help do up small buttons. Avoid clothes that are done up at the back.

Where you keep your clothes matters too. Bending down to pull open low, stiff drawers should be avoided as far as possible. So should cluttered pathways between the bed, bath or shower, chest of drawers and dressing table. Clothing should be stored in as open a way as possible – perhaps on open shelves behind a curtain.

Personal hygiene

Bathing and washing can be painful and difficult for someone suffering from arthritis. An occupational therapist can pinpoint areas where difficulties may arise and suggest simple but effective solutions. Rails on the bathroom wall are useful, and rails on the edge of the bath are vital as soon as getting in and out proves painful. A non-slip rubber mat on the bottom of the bath is a wise safety measure. Taps that have push up and down controls are easier than ones that have to be turned. If you have problems with your wrists and shoulders, a back brush may be awkward to use – opt instead for a back-scrubbing strap. Put the soap somewhere where there is no risk of slipping on it.

If your fingers are even moderately affected, you may find using an ordinary toothbrush or razor difficult. Long handles can be fitted to toothbrushes. Electric razors may be easier and safer to use than ones in plastic handles.

Getting on and off the lavatory seat can be a problem with painful knees, hips and weak legs. A higher toilet seat to reduce the distance you have to raise and lower yourself helps. It can be installed with the toilet or bought as an add-on. Arm rests can be attached to the toilet and rails can be fitted to help you get up and down. It is important to have these aids properly fitted.

Preparing and eating food

In the kitchen, store items used every day in easy-to-reach places, where you don't have to stretch or bend excessively. You may need a variety of gadgets to make your life easier. You can buy an electric can opener to open tins, for example. Corkscrews should be the double-action type that avoid the need for pulling.

Occupational therapists can advise on a range of aids for eating and drinking. Serrated knives help in cutting up food. High-friction plastic or rubber mats placed under the plates stop them from slipping around. Specially designed mugs and other utensils that are easier to grip are also available.

Find out more

Managing the pain	*138–141*
Exercise	*148–151*
Aids and gadgets	*152–153*

Removing tightly screwed lids from jars can be frustrating and painful if your fingers or wrists are even slightly affected. However, an occupational therapist can introduce you to many gadgets – including one to unscrew lids from jars – to make everyday tasks easier.

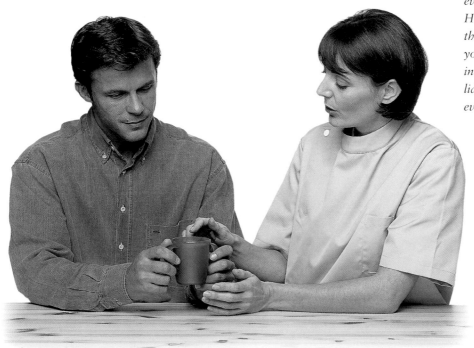

Giving up smoking

Although smoking is not a direct cause of arthritis, it is now known to be a risk factor. Smoking contributes to so many health problems, that almost any illness is more serious in smokers than in non-smokers. Some of the ill effects of smoking may be especially harmful to people with arthritis.

If you just can't give up smoking, you should seek professional help. A doctor may recommend one of the products that are available in the form of patches, chewing gums and cigarette substitutes to help wean you off your addiction gradually.

Because research has shown that many people remain surprisingly unaware of the harmful effects of smoking, and they are still vulnerable to peer-group pressure and tobacco advertising, it is worthwhile summarizing just a few of the risks here:
• People who smoke tobacco have a much greater risk of developing cancer of the lung, mouth, throat, oesophagus, bladder, kidney, pancreas and cervix.
• Smokers are more likely to develop high blood pressure, coronary heart disease and blood clots, causing bad circulation in the legs, which sometimes leads to gangrene and the need to amputate a limb. Smokers may also develop other circulatory problems.

• People affected severely by rheumatoid arthritis may develop circulatory problems. Smoking doubles the risk. Arthritis usually limits mobility and so, eventually, does smoking through the damage done to the circulatory system.

The dangerous effects of passive smoking – where a non-smoker unavoidably inhales tobacco smoke by being near someone who is smoking – have now been conclusively proved, and most people, especially parents of young children, are aware of this condition. If you do smoke, don't be surprised if you find yourself deprived of the company of children and other non-smokers.

Giving it up

It has long been known that nicotine affects the brain and causes addiction in the same way that heroin does. Although nictoine is profoundly addictive, the good news is that the habit can be kicked. There are, for example, about 11 million ex-smokers in the United Kingdom alone. You will need self-motivation before you can give up, and the first step is to consciously make the decision to stop – no one else can do this for you.

An incentive to give up smoking is to remind yourself of how expensive it is. Work out how much money you spend on smoking every year. One method to encourage yourself at the start is to set aside the money you save by not smoking and use it to treat yourself when you reach certain target days, such as a month or a year after your last cigarette.

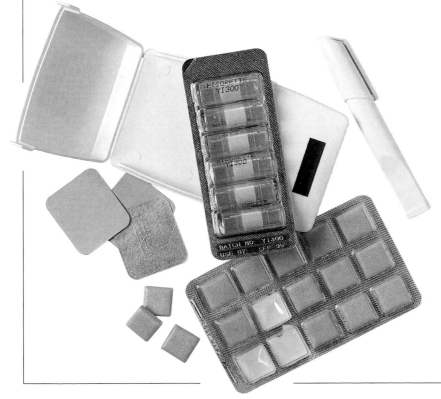

AVOIDING THE SMOKING HABIT

To help you stop smoking, go to places that do not allow smoking, such as:
- *go swimming;*
- *go to the theatre or cinema;*
- *stay the weekend with non-smoking friends;*
- *work as a hospital volunteer helper several hours a week;*
- *offer to help friends or relatives with baby sitting, where you know you cannot smoke;*
- *travel by public transport rather than by car;*
- *visit your favourite department store;*
- *go to a gym or exercise class, if your arthritis permits you;*
- *offer your services, such as helping with reading, to a local primary school.*

Quit, a charity that is devoted to helping people give up smoking, have developed these guidelines to help you stop smoking:
- Treat yourself with the money you save.
- Make a date to stop smoking and stick to it. Most people who succeed do so by stopping completely all at once, not by gradually cutting down.
- Keep busy to help you through the first few days. (Many people find that they need to keep their hands occupied.) Throw away your unopened cigarette packets, ashtrays, matches and lighters.
- Drink lots of water, perhaps with orange or lemon slices to make it more palatable. Keep a glass by you and sip from it steadily.
- Be more active, because this will help you relax. If your arthritis allows it, take the stairs instead of the lift, go for a swim or join an exercise class at your local leisure centre.
- If you suffer from withdrawal symptoms, such as irritability, nervousness, headaches or sore throats, don't worry. They are all signs that your body is readjusting to doing without the nicotine and, when that has happened, the unpleasant symptoms will stop.

- Change your routine to avoid smoking-linked activities. Take a detour so that you don't pass the shop where you used to buy your cigarettes, and above all (it is only for little while) don't go for drinks in pubs with friends who smoke.
- Don't use a celebration as an excuse for just one cigarette. Research shows that for most people, one cigarette usually leads to another.
- As time goes on, watch your weight even more carefully than you usually do. Stopping smoking sometimes increases a desire for sweet things. Although it is difficult not to be affected by this, it can be compensated for by eating a more healthy diet.
- Take it one day at a time. Each day that you don't smoke represents a real improvement in your health. Even after only a few days breathing will be more easy and energy levels will increase.

If you do lapse, don't talk yourself into believing that you have "blown it" for good. Just don't smoke any more. One or two lapses may mean that you have lost those particular battles, but you haven't lost the war.

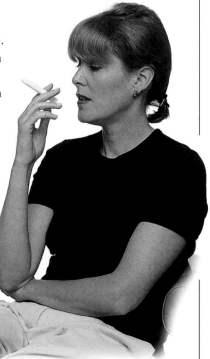

Relaxing with a cigarette in stressful times is one main reason that people fail to give up smoking – instead, find other ways to relax (see pages 58–59).

Surgery

After all other treatments have failed or proved inappropriate, surgery is sometimes the only remaining option. In some cases the arthritic joint is completely replaced but, in others, a less drastic procedure may be attempted first.

SYNOVECTOMY

Synovectomy is the surgical removal of the synovium, the thin membrane that lines the normally fluid-filled joint capsule, the cavity where the ends of two bones meet in a joint. The operation is usually performed to treat cases of severely disabling rheumatoid arthritis that have failed to respond to other treatments, which may have included injections of cortico-steroid drugs, non-steroidal anti-inflammatory drugs (NSAIDs) and other anti-rheumatic drugs.

Synovectomy is carried out to relieve chronic synovitis, inflammation of the synovium. In a normal joint the synovium secretes synovial fluid to lubricate the joint. An inflamed synovium secretes a thinner, less viscous fluid, which has inferior lubricating properties. Removing the synovium is a drastic step but it can be highly beneficial. In rheumatoid arthritis, for example, the synovium becomes diseased, so leaving it in place may eventually do more harm than good.

Rheumatoid arthritis

The synovium is the part of the body first and worst affected by rheumatoid arthritis. Synovia surround all the moveable joints of the body and rheumatoid arthritis may affect any of them – but it is much more common in some than in others. For example, the joints in the middle of the fingers and the knuckles are affected in up to 95 per cent of people with rheumatoid arthritis, whereas hip, elbow and knee joints are

affected in up to 50 per cent.

The symptoms begin with inflammation of the synovial membrane, caused by the migration of white blood cells to the membrane which, for some unknown reason, is treated by the immune system as though it were the site of a dangerous infection. The synovium often proliferates and forms "fronds" in the joint. (Some of these will be removed if a synovectomy is performed, but some will remain.) Later the tissues around the affected joint or joints, the entire synovium and, sometimes, the tendons that attach muscles to bones all become thickened by the growth of abnormal so-called pannus tissue.

Rheumatoid arthritis does not always progress this far. An attack of inflammation can often be controlled by NSAIDs. They can prevent or reduce the formation of prostaglandins, the locally acting hormones released around joints at an early stage of rheumatoid arthritis, which contribute to inflammation, swelling and pain. If NSAIDs or other treatments can be used to counter the effects of inflammation, synovitis can be controlled and surgery avoided.

Osteoarthritis

In osteoarthritis damage to the synovium may be secondary to cartilage damage. Obesity, a sudden blow, or a gradual accumulation of damage caused by a job or a way of life that puts constant and unnatural strain on joints can all contribute to the breakdown of cartilage that causes the symptoms of osteoarthritis.

The breakdown causes the surface of the cartilage to become ragged and pockmarked. As the cartilage deteriorates, the ends of the bones that are normally cushioned by it may begin to rub together. The body may respond to this by producing more cartilage than normal to try to fill the gap, but the extra cartilage is usually of inferior quality and lacks the shock-absorbing properties of normal cartilage.

Synovectomy is rarely used for treating osteoarthritis.

How the operation is performed

Synovectomy may be performed under general anaesthetic when the joint is opened and the abnormal tissue cut away and removed. Increasingly, synovectomy is performed using keyhole surgery techniques, in which the synovium is removed through a small hole using a special instrument called an arthroscope. The use of an arthroscope reduces time spent in hospital. The removal of the synovium sounds a drastic procedure, but the human body is remarkably adaptable and, with the removal of the worst affected tissue, the joint may perform surprisingly well.

DEBRIDEMENT

Debridement comes from a French word meaning "tidying up". It is used when the load-bearing surfaces and the lining of the joint have become worn or damaged, so that small portions fall off, get into the joint and cause swelling. Where there is a mechanical problem, such as a worn weight-bearing surface, debridement can be useful. In the treatment of arthritis about 95 per cent of such operations are done on the knee, because that

is the joint that is most vulnerable to this kind of damage. The majority of debridements today are performed with an arthroscope which enables the surgeon to see into the joint, using keyhole surgery which means that only a tiny incision is necessary.

A normal joint's bearing surface should be a smooth, white glistening surface. An abnormal joint surface looks like crab meat, with little white bits sticking up in the air. The idea is to smooth the bearing surfaces of the joint. The inside of the joint is inspected through the arthroscope and anything that is rough or uneven is trimmed back, using a surgical power tool. The operation to smooth it down is sometimes applied to bone as well as to cartilage.

The operation involves a general or – sometimes – local anaesthetic. Usually patients will not be in hospital for more than a day. They will have some swelling afterward but will probably be able to walk quite soon.

What can you expect?

The results of debridement are generally good, but they tend not to last long. It is usually performed on patients in their 40s or early 50s who are moving toward joint replacement. It may postpone the need for joint replacement by 18 months or two years or even longer, but the symptoms of joint damage will usually return. It may be possible to perform a second debridement, but each time the operation is performed the period of relief is shorter.

Debridement is a holding operation carried out on slightly worn joints in order to postpone more serious surgery. As time goes on and joint replacements continue to improve, the need for debridement will increasingly disappear.

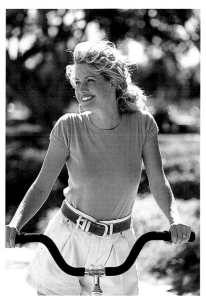

After a debridement operation, young patients are expected to do non-impact exercises to build strength. Cycling, swimming or rowing are all suitable, but jogging is not advised for some time afterward.

Surgery

OSTEOTOMY

The need for osteotomy – the word simply means cutting a bone – can arise when the joint involving the bone is not in the right position.

Essentially, osteotomy involves cutting a bone so that it can be put back in a different position. This procedure is sometimes necessary in the hip, often in the knee, frequently in the foot and rarely in other joints. It may also be performed after a fracture when bones have not healed in the right position; in this case the surgeon may choose to cut the bones so that they can be realigned to heal in the correct position.

Who can it help?

An osteotomy may be performed on the hip if a person is born with a hip joint that lies in the wrong place. In such cases the top end of the thigh bone may be a little too straight, so that the ball of the ball-and-socket joint slips out of the joint sideways – this is referred to by surgeons as "uncovered". The osteotomy involves breaking the top end of the thigh bone, bending it in and resetting it. It is then put back in the socket (known technically as acetabulum of the hip). This is the most common use of osteotomy performed on large bones.

Osteotomy of the knee may be used on patients in an older age group, usually because the patient has been bow-legged, a condition present since childhood. (This was often due to rickets, caused by a deficiency of vitimin D; this is now rare.) This results in more weight than is desirable being carried by one side of the joint, which may, consequently, become excessively worn.

An orthopaedic surgeon can often solve the problem by breaking the shin bone – or the tibia – taking a wedge out of it and joining it again. This procedure allows the weight to be transferred from the worn side of the knee joint to the unworn side.

Smaller joints are sometimes a candidate for an osteotomy. The most common such application is for the bones of the foot. The metatarsals, the bones between the ankle and the base of the toes, sometimes drop down so that those people affected feel as if they are walking on stones around the base of their toes. The operation to correct this condition simply involves breaking or cutting the bones and resetting them, so the hard ends that have been pressing on the ground can ride up.

What can I expect?

Like any broken bone that has been reset, an osteotomy will take approximately four to six weeks to heal. The results of this operation in the short term are generally good, but as with most other types of surgery, they are hard to guarantee. The average duration of relief from symptoms is from 7 to 10 years. Afterward an operation for the replacement of a hip or knee joint is usually required.

With the increasing use of joint replacements and a growing ability to correct abnormalities early without resorting to surgery, osteotomies are less common today than they once were, but the technique remains valuable in certain cases. An osteotomy is normally carried out under general anaesthetic.

Osteotomies do not usually need to be repeated. Sometimes the bone needs to be stabilized in its new position by a metal plate to hold it in place, in which case the patient may have to stay in hospital for up to two weeks. But normally patients can leave the hospital within a few days.

ARTHRODESIS

An operation in which a joint is cut out altogether, and the cut ends of the bones that used to meet in the joint are fused together is known as an arthrodesis. This is an effective, although drastic, way of removing severe pain in a joint affected by arthritis. It completely removes all diseased tissue and eliminates the possibility of further arthritis in that area.

When surgical techniques were less developed than they are now, arthrodesis was the treatment for many cases of rheumatoid arthritis and osteoarthritis. The operation was first widely used to treat cases of tuberculosis, which affected joints and made them stiff and sore. The disease itself sometimes caused the joint to fuse and the pain to go, so surgeons took to doing the same thing artificially.

Who might benefit?

Today, arthrodesis is used only rarely in severe osteoarthritis, in cases in which the pain is so severe and the crippling effect so considerable that the price paid in loss of mobility or freedom of movement is considered worth paying. The joint most commonly removed by arthrodesis today is the big toe, to get rid of a bunion, a form of osteoarthritis in which the joint is severely deformed by wear and tear.

If you are not particularly young or athletic, arthrodesis or fusion, the other name given to this operation, is not a high price to pay for permanent freedom from the pain of a bunion. Arthrodesis can make your walking a bit stiff and awkward, although most people become used to this condition.

Very occasionally, after major injuries

or major infections, it may be necessary to perform arthrodesis of the knee, or – very rarely – of the hip. This cuts out the infection completely and gets rid of the pain; however, it also causes a major disability, by making the leg into a straight, inflexible rigid structure, or fusing the leg to the hip.

People who have had the operation performed, usually learn to walk well. The biggest social disadvantage tends to be in travelling, because of the problems in tucking a rigid leg out of the way in a car, train or airplane, especially in crowded conditions.

In spite of these problems, arthrodesis may be the best solution for rapidly progressive rheumatoid arthritis in a very young person, for whom it is too early to perform a joint replacement, or in an elderly patient whose first or possibly second joint replacement has failed, and for whom there is little or no chance of success with a further replacement.

Arthrodesis can be used in the fingers and in the ankles. It is sometimes used to fuse the two top vertebrae of the neck damaged by arthritis.

Arthrodesis requires a general anaesthetic. How long a stay in hospital it involves will depend upon whether or not the fixed joint needs to be stabilized – held together – while it fuses. Occasionally, depending on where and how it was performed, it may be possible to reverse an arthrodesis and to recreate the joint that has been removed in such an operation.

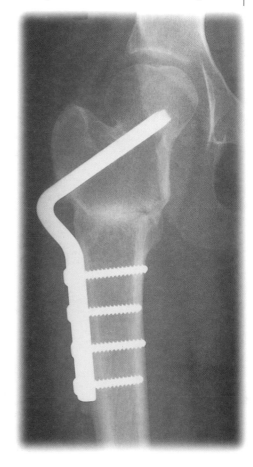

This X-ray was taken after a femoral osteotomy to treat osteoarthritis of the hip. The femur (thigh bone) was cut directly below the joint, and the two ends of the bone realigned with metal fixation screwed to the femur, in much the same way as if the femur had been broken accidentally.

Joint replacement

The history of joint replacement dates from 1891 when German surgeons experimented with an ivory ball-and-socket hip joint fixed to bone with nickel-plated screws. Today there are a number of different types of artificial hip joints, and many thousands of them are fitted every year all over the world.

The most common reason that a joint deteriorates enough to consider a replacement joint is osteoarthritis; but it may also be helpful in treating joint disease caused by rheumatoid arthritis. Your doctor will take into consideration the amount of your pain you suffer and the measure of your disability, and if these are having serious effects on your quality of life and daily activities.

If a replacement surgery is recommended, this should not depress you: if the decision is properly considered, these operations are usually very successful. You will be given strong warnings to not expect a complete change. However, they often accompany a replacement surgery because people who receive a new joint often experience a great improvement in their quality of life. The new freedom of movement and absence of pain often make them believe that they can do anything, and they can expect too much from their new joint.

To the enormous numbers of people who yearly gain relief from grinding, inescapable severe pain, joint replacement often seems like a miracle. The fact that such operations may be performed on people who are in their 90s is a measure of the confidence that surgeons now have in this operation.

Replacing the hip joint

This type of replacement is one of the great surgical success stories, and only someone who has experienced the relief it can bring can really appreciate what it means. Standard replacement hip joints take the form of a metallic ball, usually made of a chromium or titanium metal alloy, with a long spike attached to one

Cartilage layer

Femoral head

Femur

Metal cup

Metal head

Plastic cup

Metal ball joint

Femoral hip prosthesis

THE HIP JOINT

When the cartilage on the femur and the socket of the pelvic bone (far left) deteriorates, surgery may be required to repair the joint. A new, less invasive method uses a metal cup and metal head to resurface the socket and femur (centre). The standard method uses a metal ball and plastic cup.

end. The socket on the pelvis in which the ball naturally rotates is replaced by a socket made of extremely high density polyethylene plastic.

Under general anaesthetic, incisions are made into the pelvic area. To gain access to the bones, the surrounding muscles are either pushed away or cut. The joint must then be dislocated. The natural bone ball at the top of the femur is removed and a shaft is driven deep into the femur to take the metal spike. The socket in the pelvis is enlarged to accept the new artificial socket. A special type of cement is used to hold both the spike and socket in place. After the ball is positioned in the socket, any muscle and tendon repair work necessary is performed and the incisions are closed.

A second replacement surgery

The very success of hip replacement surgery has brought with it new problems. Hip replacements are being fitted in increasingly younger people because of the enhanced quality of life they can provide. However, this means that artificial joints are wearing out well before death (the average life of a new joint is 10–15 years), so there is a growing need for second joint replacements.

Although a second hip replacement continues to leave the person involved free from pain and much more mobile than they would be without the operation, the results are never as good as for a first operation. The second operation has to be performed on a patient who is older and more frail and, therefore, that much less suitable to face the slight but real risks of major surgery.

The future of joint replacement

Scientists and engineers are currently trying to produce a hip replacement that will last substantially longer than those in use today. Although some prostheses have been shown to be defective, until recently the main reason why the joints failed was that the spike driven into the femur gradually became loose; improved cements have largely solved this problem.

This colour-enhanced X-ray shows the metal spike and plastic socket of a hip replacement.

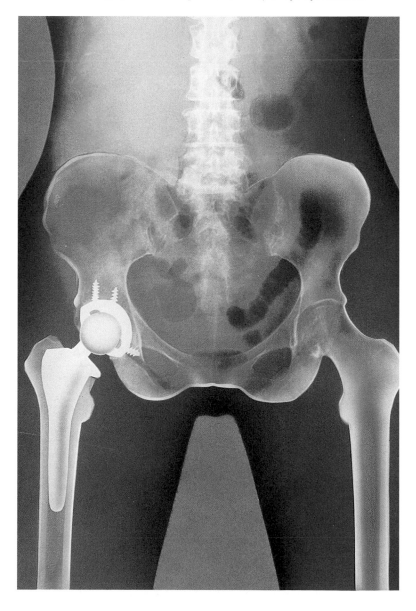

Joint replacement

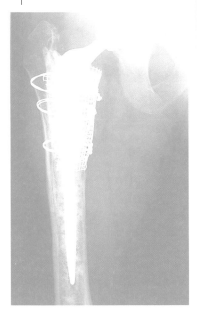

A total hip replacement can be seen in this X-ray. The femur (thigh bone) was cut to accommodate the metal shaft, and the pelvis was drilled to take the socket. A metal cage held in place with wires surrounds the upper portion of the joint. Small pieces of bone from the femoral head were placed in the cage to help fuse the bone component.

The next set of problems are those caused by wear of the joint, and especially wear of the surface of the polyethylene cup in which the ball rotates. The debris released as this plastic surface is gradually worn down causes a biological reaction, which weakens the surrounding bone and steadily weakens the joint.

Scientists are tackling this problem in different ways. A new experimental prosthesis uses only metal components to resurface the femur head and the socket in the pelvis. It is suitable for younger patients and the bone must be of good quality, so women with osteoporosis are not candidates for the procedure.

Another promising procedure being researched by a British team involves a material similar to diamond, a hard form of carbon which could be used to coat the surfaces of artificial joints. This material has the remarkable property of being nearly as hard as diamond (and, therefore, resistant to wear) but also of being slippery and a good lubricant, like graphite, another form of carbon.

The research team is studying the effects of coating first the ball and then the socket of an artificial hip joint with the new material. They have also found that the carbon coating can be fastened securely to the lining of the natural socket, and that it does not cause any harmful biological reaction during the course of its use. This type of joint is still experimental, but it may extend the lives of hip joints by 5 to 10 years.

Before the operation

If you decide to have a joint replacement operation – the final decision will, of course, be yours – you will usually be invited to attend a pre-operation clinic or other session, at which you will be able to put questions about the operation to a specialist. You will be examined to ensure that you are sufficiently fit for the operation. You will also be advised if you need to lose weight or do any more exercise than you are doing already.

You will probably be admitted to hospital the day before your operation – possibly earlier if you have any condition that requires special attention such as a heart condition. On the day of the operation you will be given a pill or injection to relax you. In the operating theatre you will be given either a general anaesthetic or a local one to make you lose all feeling below the waist. If the latter is elected, you will also be given sedatives during the operation.

Recovering from surgery

An intravenous drip – a tube in a vein in your arm which is used to supply fluid and any necessary medication directly to your bloodstream – will be left in place after the operation. You will also find one or two tubes coming out of your hip. These remove the fluid produced as the body heals after the surgery.

You will be taken to a recovery room or high-level care unit, and stay there until the doctors feel your condition is stable. You will then be taken back to your ward. You will probably have a pad or pillow fixed between your legs to hold them apart and in the right position. You will be given painkillers to help relieve pain after the operation.

Drips and drains are often removed 24 to 48 hours after the operation. You will be encouraged to walk as soon as possible after that, as moderate exercise speeds healing and improves health. You will probably walk first with a frame and then with sticks.

CASE HISTORY

Richard Dewing, who is 61 years old, had had recurrent pain around his back for several years.

"At first I didn't think my hips had anything to do with it, but as it got worse I was given more painkillers. I finally went to an osteopath, and he was the first person to suggest that a hip operation might be beneficial. I was at first rather cynical and felt I was a bit young – I was then 55 – but I went to see a surgeon who took X-rays.

When I saw them the joints looked absolutely horrible. The balls of the ball and socket joints looked terribly ragged and the whole joint looked jagged. Both hips looked equally disastrous. My general practitioner was very enthusiastic that surgery was my best option, and I had great confidence in my surgeon, who explained the operation to me. So I decided to have my hips done.

The first thing I noticed after the first operation was the quite extraordinary relief from pain in the replaced hip – pain which I had hardly associated with the hip. It is not easy to know what's going on in that region, but it used to hurt in a very nasty way and the pain could shoot off down the legs and around the place. But by about two days after the operation it definitely felt better, and I couldn't wait to have the other one done. In fact there was a six to eight month gap.

At the time just before the first hip was done I couldn't walk very far

because it hurt to walk. I had to have high seats to sit on and I was looking around for handles to pull myself up on. A lot of things in life had become very uncomfortable and a lot of jobs had become very difficult. Now, a few years after my second operation, I can do a lot of things that I couldn't do before: walk miles, run if I have to, though it is not recommended, sit on anything and not just carefully chosen high chairs, cut my own toenails and do up shoelaces – which is a great relief.

I'd advise anyone whose doctor thinks they would definitely benefit from hip replacement to go for it. It's a routine operation with very slight risks attached; it relieves bad pain which is terribly important and it changes one's life for the better. It's very rejuvenating."

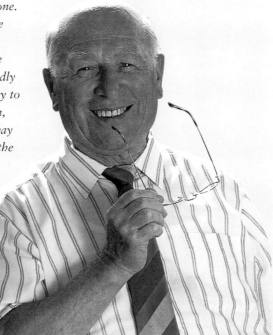

Joint replacement

Knee replacements

The success of the first total hip joint replacement has led to the development of other replacement joints. The knee is the second most common joint to be replaced.

Most people with arthritis in their knees will never need a replacement joint. Although surgery is available for those that do, a doctor will be more conservative in recommending one because the artificial joints have been available for a shorter period than artificial hip joints, and inserting them requires more complex surgery.

Unlike the ball-and-socket hip joint, which needs to rotate in various directions, the knee was thought to move mainly in one direction. Early knee replacements were simple hinges, held together with a pin. However, it became clear that, as well as moving on a hinge, the natural knee joint does rotate slightly, so the one-dimensional movement typical of early knee replacements soon had a limited life. Today, a number of different knee replacement designs are available to suit the needs of different patients.

Knee surgery

If you agree that you need a replacement and both your knees are affected, it may be possible to have both done together. However, bear in mind that recovery usually goes more smoothly if one is done before the other, and that one knee is often considerably worse affected than the other, so two successive operations are usually desirable.

The general procedure before and after the operation is similar to that for a hip replacement. After the operation you may be asked to start moving your new joint within two or three days or not for a week or two, depending upon the type of joint you have had fitted.

Later on you may asked to use a passive exerciser, which bends and straightens your knee independently of your movement. You may be walking on your new joint in only two or three weeks; however, you may have to wait longer if cement holding it in place requires more time to set.

The great majority of those who receive new knees are delighted with the

The artificial components used to repair a knee joint are highlighted in this colour-enhanced X-ray.

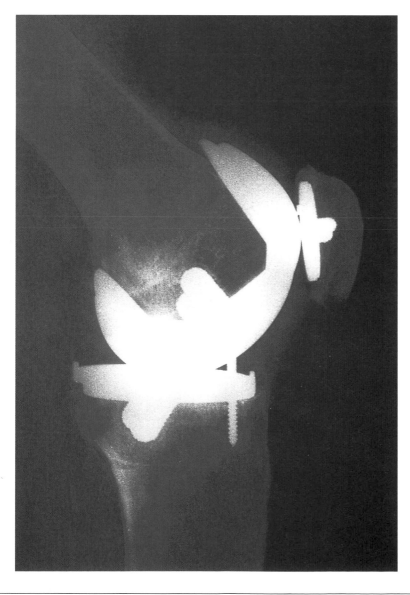

final outcome. Your new knee joint will give you good relief from pain, and after you've recuperated from the operation, you will have sufficient freedom of movement for most activities.

Other joint replacements

Knuckle joints are now routinely replaced. More experimentally, the shoulder and elbow are also being replaced. In addition, rapid progress is being made at present with the design of new finger- and ankle-joint replacements.

Leaving hospital

How fast you can return to normal life after an operation – which will almost certainly be a better life than before the procedure – depends on a number of factors: your age, the type of joint replaced, the condition of your other joints and what sort of shape your muscles are in.

Most people are able to leave hospital within 6 to 10 days, although there may be special circumstances that will require a longer stay. While you will have relief from the joint pain, be careful that you don't over-do things. You will need to take special care for the first 8 to 12 weeks after your operation as you get used to your new way of life.

What you can and can't do

Your physiotherapist and occupational therapist, and/or your doctor, will supply you with a list of things that you must not do with a replacement joint. It is vital that you follow these instructions precisely. What you can and cannot do will depend on the type of joint fitted and your individual case.

It is vital to remember that an artificial hip joint is never as good as the natural joint. You will be advised if you have a replacement hip joint, for example, to avoid too much bending at the hips. You will also be told, and this is more difficult to remember, not to cross your legs because that can dislocate your new hip, which is not held in place as firmly as the natural one.

Your physiotherapist will help you with an individual program of exercises, which will be tailored to suit you and to strengthen your muscles. You will be able to walk, swim (avoiding breaststroke because of the effort required by hips and knees) and ride a bicycle. You should avoid running and playing games on hard surfaces – these can jar and overload the joint. Most kinds of moderate exercise, however, are good for you and your new joint is designed to cope with them.

You will probably be able to drive a car again after four to six weeks, but be advised not to bend your hips or raise your legs too much as you get in and out.

WHAT ARE THE RISKS?

Joint replacement, especially hip replacement, is routine surgery, but there is a small risk of complications with any operation. Blood clots may form and dislodge, often ending up in the lungs; this is rare but if it happens, it can cause blockages in blood vessels in the lungs, breathlessness, collapse and even death.

On rare occasions the area around a joint can become infected. In this case the replacement components may have to be removed while the infection is treated. The components are then reimplanted several weeks later.

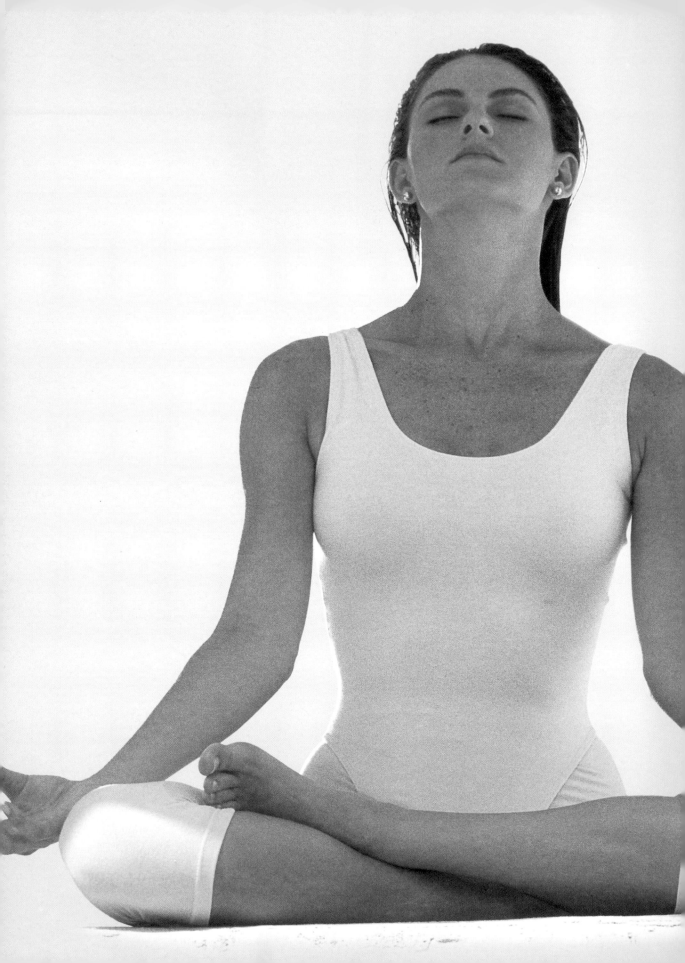

4

LIVING WITH

ARTHRITIS

Arthritis is a challenge, both physically and emotionally. When you realize that it has become part of your life you may feel depressed, with a lack of appetite and poor sleep, and be anxious about your future and your ability to care for yourself. But you can cope with arthritis if you take control, rather than let it control you. This means learning about the condition, finding ways around physical limitations, being open with family and friends, and setting goals that you can realistically achieve.

There are ways to boost and maintain your health and this chapter will help you confront the psychological and physical challenges.

Managing the pain

One of the biggest challenges facing people with arthritis is pain. The degree of pain can vary; sometimes it's worse than at other times. However, there are many other ways besides drugs that can help ease the pain. What works for one person may not do the trick for another, so you may have to try out several methods.

Pain in arthritis

Sensations of pain vary widely among people with arthritis – as do the things that provoke or relief them. What makes you feel pain is inflammation in the joint areas, causing swelling, redness, local heat and loss of movement. Damaged or worn joints can be painful, too. Both of these can lead to the pain of muscle strain caused by trying to protect the joints from painful movements.

Left untreated, pain can sap your energy and leave you virtually unable to function. It can make you feel angry and full of self-pity. You will have to acknowledge pain as a fact of life, but if you give in to pain it can have a

destructive effect, affecting your mood, outlook and relationships. If you are anxious, depressed, stressed or fatigued the pain feels worse. If you are not careful, you can be caught in a vicious circle of pain, depression and stress which can interfere with your quality of life. But, when you learn to manage your pain, this is less likely to happen.

Natural pain relievers

The brain and spinal cord can release their own pain-relieving chemicals, called endorphins, and these have a similar chemical structure to the powerful, pain-killing drug known as morphine. You can help release the endorphins in

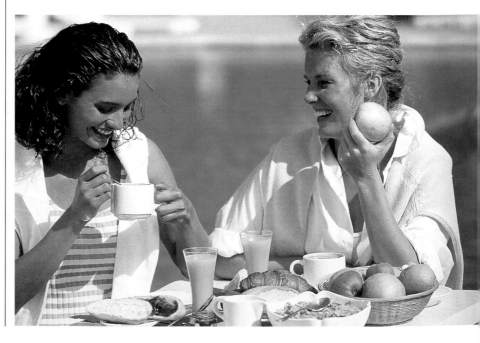

Enjoying a healthy and happy lifestyle will help you to stay in a positive frame of mind.

HELPFUL THERAPIES

One of the great strengths of the complementary therapies is their ability to relieve pain. Turn now to:

* *T'ai chi*   *(page 48–49)*
* *Herbalism*   *(page 82–85)*
* *Homeopathy*   *(page 86–89)*

* *Osteopathy*   *(page 90–91)*
* *Chiropractic*   *(page 92–93)*
* *Reflexology*   *(page 96–99)*

your body by exercising – for example, the runner's "high" is the result of endorphins being released – as well as with massage, heat, cold, hydrotherapy, physiotherapy, sex and a positive attitude.

A positive attitude to pain

Keeping a positive attitude means that you are less likely to lead a life that revolves around pain and illness. The occasional moan and groan is to be expected, but the more you get locked into pain the worse it can feel. Try and take your mind off the pain by doing the things that you like – enjoy humour, eat good food, do some exercise every day, go out with friends. Give yourself treats and have something to look forward to every day. Indulge yourself and go to bed each night in a good frame of mind.

    Recommended techniques to combat stress and fatigue include regular exercise, relaxation, saying "No" so that you don't take on too much, getting enough rest, pacing yourself, keeping a good body posture and getting enough sleep.

Protecting your joints

You can protect your joints by doing daily activities in ways that reduce stress on your joints.
* Become aware of your body's positions and avoid activities that involve a tight

grip or put too much pressure on your fingers. Avoid holding one position for a long time.
* Use your largest and strongest joints and muscles for daily tasks wherever possible. Spread the weight of an object over many joints to reduce the stress on any one joint.
* Use aids and gadgets to make difficult tasks easier (see pages 152–153).
* Control your weight to avoid extra stress on your weight-bearing joints and further pain and joint damage (see pages 116–117).
* Ask for help when you need it. Don't suffer in silence.

Saving energy

* Listen to your body for signals that it needs to rest.
* Pace yourself, don't push yourself. If you overdo things it can lead to exhaustion and could cause a flare-up.
* Don't expend energy on things that really don't matter. Look at ways of doing things that involve the least energy expenditure.
* Try to achieve a healthy balance between activity and rest. Sit down when you can and plan rest times for when you know you will be able to take them, but don't rest too much as this can cause muscle stiffness.

Managing the pain

MANAGING PAIN WITHOUT DRUGS

HEAT

Heat methods are best for joints and soft tissues with long-standing arthritis. **Moist Heat:** Soak in a nice hot bath. Add oils or Epsom salts. • There are several manufacturers of home-spa equipment which is recommended for arthritis. You lie on a special mattress connected by a hose to a machine which blows air, making the water bubble. • Put warm towels or hot packs where you need them. You should not do this for longer than 15 to 20 minutes three times a day.
Dry Heat: Heating pads can be used to warm painful areas. Some just need to be popped in a microwave oven to heat up. • Electric blankets and mattress pads are very comforting. • Flannelette sheets feel warmest against the skin. • A hot water bottle wrapped in a towel keeps selected parts of the body warm. • Warming clothes on the radiator before you put them on can help. • Deep-heat massagers provide deep heat inside the joint but with no risk of burning the skin.

COLD

Cold, best for the acute inflammation of joints during a flare-up, reduces swelling, lessens muscle spasms and numbs pain. Buy a cold pack from a chemist, or make your own by wrapping a damp cloth or towel around a bag of frozen vegetables. Apply for 10 to 15 minutes at a time. Do not use if you have poor circulation.

CONTRAST BATH

Contrast bath: this is a combined hot and cold treatment. You soak a hand or foot in warm water, then cold, then warm again.

HYDROTHERAPY

Water therapy removes the pull of gravity, allowing you to do gentle exercises to reduce stiffness and decrease pain in your joints. Many health farms have warm spa baths and pools that are invigorating and relaxing. Hydrotherapy is a standard treatment available at a number of physiotherapy centres. Exercises or aquarobics at your local swimming pool are also good for arthritis. (See also pages 66–67.)

MASSAGE

Massage involves massaging or kneading the muscles in a painful area to increase the blood flow and bring warmth. You may be able to do this yourself. If not, ask a partner or close friend, or find a professional masseur. Using an oil can help hands glide over the skin, and some people find that using a lubrication eases pain. If pain develops while having a massage, stop. Do not massage a joint that is already inflamed. (See also pages 68–71.)

DEEP-HEAT RUBS

Also known as rubefacients or counter-irritants, these block the sensation of pain and increase local bloodflow in the skin.

SPLINTS

Splints rest the joint, so reducing inflammation and pain. They should be used with caution since they can cause joints to become weak.

MANAGING PAIN WITHOUT DRUGS

TENS	TENS (transcutaneous electrical nerve stimulation) involves stimulation of the nerves by low-level electrical impulses (see pages 120-121). It does not hurt, but it may cause tingling. TENS is particularly helpful for treating localized pain.
COPPER BRACELET	One research study suggests that by wearing a copper bracelet, minute amounts of copper transfer through the skin, relieving pain and stiffness. The benefits of this traditional remedy are controversial.
RELAXATION THERAPY	Relaxation calms mind and body and releases tension in your muscles, so relieving pain. You need a quiet place and 20 minutes to yourself. Play some music or listen to natural sounds such as water. Find a comfortable position, breathe deeply, think tranquil thoughts and imagine pleasant scenes. You feel calm, refreshed and with a renewed sense of wellbeing. Other forms of relaxation involve guided imagery or visualization, where a voice on tape guides you through a beautiful scene. (See also pages 58–59.)
MEDITATION	Some say meditation makes them feel refreshed and revitalized. It quietens the mind and lessens stress, thus reducing pain. You can meditate with a mantra, by focusing on breathing, or by concentrating on a small object such as a flower. (See also pages 54–55.) Some people find prayer relaxing and comforting.
HYPNOSIS	Hypnosis can soothe pain by creating a state of deep relaxation so that you can accept suggestions for positive change. (See also pages 60–61).
SLEEP	A good night's sleep restores energy and increases your ability to manage pain. It also gives your joints a chance to rest. Make sure that you go to bed at about the same time every night and invest in a comfortable bed.
ACUPUNCTURE AND ACUPRESSURE	Needles or pressure are placed at particular points, stimulating deep sensory nerves that tell the brain to release pain-killing endorphins. (See pages 78–81.)
AROMATHERAPY	Essential oils are used with massage to calm and soothe: rosemary, benzoin, German camomile, camphor, juniper or lavender do this. Cypress, fennel, lemon and wintergreen detoxify and may reduce inflammation. (See also pages 50–53.)
NUTRITIONAL THERAPY	There is evidence that the human body uses omega-3 essential fatty acids to produce prostraglandins, chemicals that can help reduce the inflammation associated with arthritis. Oily fish, such as herring, mackerel, salmon and trout, are an excellent source of these fatty acids. (See also pages 64–65 and 142–147.)

Diet

*D*oct*ers are now taking diet seriously because in recent years there has been an increasing amount of evidence that nutrition plays an important part in arthritis, particularly in rheumatoid arthritis. Research shows that changing what you eat can help relieve symptoms.*

You may not be able to cure rheumatoid arthritis with diet, but it can mean less pain, shorter periods of stiffness, and a stronger grip. Some people who change their diet are able to reduce drugs. There are some people, however, who do not benefit much by changing their diet.

Many people with rheumatoid arthritis are not eating a healthy diet. According to the journal *Arthritis and Rheumatism*, only 6 per cent of sufferers consume the recommended daily intake of selenium, which helps protect against arthritis, and only 23 per cent eat enough calcium, which is essential for strong bones. The best way of ensuring that you get these and other essential nutrients is to eat a healthy, balanced diet.

Being overweight can make symptoms of arthritis worse. The most important thing that you can do is to lose weight. Eating a balanced diet and taking exercise (see pages 148–151) will help you to do so.

Many people with arthritis can relieve their symptoms with a combination of healthy dietary changes and medication.

What is a balanced diet?

Start by increasing your intake of starchy foods, which contain complex carbohydrates, and fresh fruit and vegetables. Complex carbohydrates are digested more slowly, providing energy over a longer period than refined carbohydrates such as sugar. Ideally, two-thirds of your calories should come from complex carbohydrates, which are found in pasta, grains and vegetables.

Eat a multi-coloured range of fresh fruit and vegetables to get a mixture of nutrients. Cooking vegetables by steaming or microwaving them is the best way to retain their nutrients. Try to eat at least one totally vegetarian meal once a week. When eating meat, choose mainly from poultry sources.

Cut down on your fat intake – fat has twice the number of calories as protein and carbohydrates. Saturated fats, found in biscuits, cheese, margarine, pastry and chips, are the most important type to reduce. Also reduce your sugar intake, which provides calories but not nutrients.

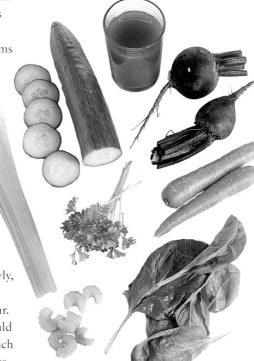

EATING FOR ARTHRITIS

Find out more
Dietary supplements 146–147
Herbal medicine   82–85

HEALTHY FOODS

FISH AND SEAFOOD	Except for gout sufferers (see pages 24–25), all fish are good, especially cold water, oily fish such as mackerel, sardines, herring, salmon, halibut, trout and tuna. Eat at least five fish meals a week.
CHICKEN, TURKEY, VEAL	Eat these instead of red meat (don't eat turkey skin).
VEGETABLES AND FRUIT	All vegetables are good, but choose especially green, leafy fresh vegetables. All fruit is fine.
WHOLE GRAINS	Wholegrain bread and brown rice are high in fibre.
POLYUNSATURATED OILS	Found in oils made from seeds such as sunflower and safflower, which contain the essential fatty acid alpha-linolenic. Add linseeds, sunflower seeds and unrefined oils to your diet.

FOODS TO AVOID

FATS AND FRIED FOOD	This category includes red meat such as beef and pork. Some recent studies have indicated that some fats can have an inflammatory effect on people who have rheumatoid arthritis.
PULSES	Some pulses, such as lentils, contain a substance called lectin, which can aggravate arthritis symptoms.
DAIRY PRODUCTS	These include milk, cheese, yoghurt, cream, dairy ice cream and other milk products. Recent studies have shown that milk products can make the symptoms of rheumatoid arthritis and psoriatic arthritis worse in some people.
FIZZY DRINKS	The phospates in fizzy drinks deplete calcium levels.
ADDITIVES AND PERSERVATIVES	Recent research has found that, in some people, food colourings may worsen the conditions of rheumatoid arthritis and psoriatic arthritis.

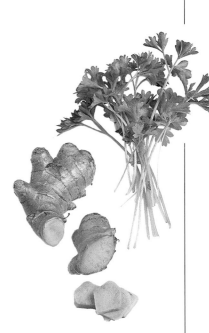

Preparing meals with certain herbs, such as ginger, which is an anti-inflammatory, and parsley, which is rich in calcium, have been found to be useful in the treatment of arthritis.

CHAPTER FOUR

Diet

Most people realize that there are very real benefits in maintaining a good diet. As an arthritis sufferer, it is especially important to realize you can effect real improvement in your condition by being careful of what you eat.

Although people with arthritis are following a balanced, nutritious diet, they may have to take supplements to increase certain nutrients, particularly calcium and iron. Some people may also become sensitive to certain foods in their diet.

Osteoarthritis and calcium

Having a good intake of foods containing calcium from an early age to build healthy bones is thought to be the best way to prevent osteoarthritis. Your calcium needs will depend on whether you are male or female, your age, and if you are a woman, if you're pregnant or breastfeeding. The average adult over 19 years old needs 700 mg daily. Discuss with your doctor whether calcium supplements will be necessary for you.

Adequate amounts of vitamin D, needed for calcium absorption, are also required to prevent osteoporosis. This vitamin can be found in oily fish, egg yolk and some breakfast cereals, and light-skinned people can obtain it by

exposing their skin to 15 minutes of sun. Foods that inhibit calcium absorption, such as fizzy drinks, spinach and bran, should be avoided.

Why iron is important

Anaemia is often associated with arthritis, either caused by having a chronic disease or long-term use of non-steroidal anti-inflammatory drugs (NSAIDs). Some good sources of iron are oily fish such as sardines, pulses such as haricot beans and lentils, and dark, leafy vegetables such as spinach.

Including foods high in vitamin C (found in fruit and vegetables) will help your body asborb iron. Tea reduces the amount of iron that your body can absorb, so avoid it half an hour before and after eating a meal.

Food sensitivity

People with gout are sensitive to foods containing purine, and some researchers believe that food sensitivities can increase the symptoms of rheumatoid arthritis. Although people with this disease do not display the classic allergy reactions to particular foods, many develop symptoms when they eat them and stop getting symptoms when they do not. When you are sensitive to particular foods, the body's immune response is altered. Food sensitivities can also develop when you eat the same foods every day.

Foods that may cause a problem include eggs, nuts and seeds, onions, chocolate and members of the nightshade family, which include tomatoes, white potatoes, peppers and aubergines – and tobacco. One way to find out which foods aggravate your arthritis is to keep a diary of what you eat and note whether you experience pain, discomfort, swelling

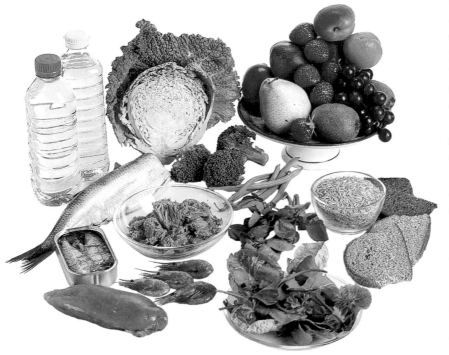

Find out more
Dietary supplements 146–147
Herbal medicine   82–85

GOOD SOURCES OF CALCIUM

The calcium found in dairy products are better absorbed than calcium from other foods; however, other foods, especially those listed here, are still useful sources of calcium.

Dairy sources

Typical serving	Calcium content (mg)
Yoghurt, 140 gml (5 oz)	240
Skimmed milk, 190 ml (⅓ pt)	236
Semi-skimmed milk, 190 ml (⅓ pt)	231
Whole milk, 190 ml (⅓ pt)	225
Cheddar cheese, 28g (1 oz)	202–207
Double gloucester cheese, 28 g (1 oz)	186
Ice cream, 112 g (4 oz)	134
Cottage cheese, 112 g (4 oz)	67

Non-dairy sources

Typical serving	Calcium content (mg)
Sardines in sauce (with bones), 56 g (2 oz)	220–258
Trout (grilled), 100 g (3½ oz)	218
Prawns (shelled), 84 g (3 oz)	126
Almonds (raw, shelled), 56 g (2 oz)	90
Spring greens (cooked), 112 g (4 oz)	84
Orange (large)	70
Baked beans, 112 g (4 oz)	60
Salmon (tinned), 56 g (2 oz)	52
Dried apricots, 56 g (2 oz)	52
Broccoli (cooked), 112 g (4 oz)	45
Spring cabbage, 112 g (4 oz)	34
Peanuts (plain), 56 g (2 oz)	34
Wholemeal bread, 60 g (2 slices)	32
Watercress, 14 g (½ oz)	31

or stiffness afterward. Some practitioners use other methods to test for food sensitivities, but these have not proven to be reliable.

Once you have identified the foods that you think may be causing symptoms, you can cut them from your diet for a month, then reintroduce them one by one to see whether or not your symptoms return. It is the only accurate and reliable way to confirm reactions to foods. Because reintroducing certain foods can cause a severe reaction, an elimination diet should be supervised by your doctor.

The naturopathic diet

For rheumatoid arthritis, naturopaths recommend a diet that is high in whole grains, vegetables and fibre, and low in sugar, animal-derived foods and refined carbohydrates.

Fasting and partial fasting

Fasting may reduce disease activity in rheumatoid arthritis and is sometimes used to good effect during flare-ups, suggesting that food may play a part in aggravating the condition. Fasting is supposed to promote health because it gives all the organs of the body a complete rest; toxins are eliminated, the system cleansed and the liver activated. Fasting changes the blood chemistry, slowing down the action of certain enzymes and blocking key steps in the chain of events that lead to inflammation and pain. Fasting is common in naturopathic and Ayurvedic medicine.

In a partial fast, you can have things such as herbal teas or fruit juices. People are sometimes put on a partial fast for around 7 to 10 days to clean out the system before starting an elimination diet.

Diet

DIETARY SUPPLEMENTS FOR RHEUMATOID ARTHRITIS

FISH OILS	Fish oils contain important fatty acids, called EPA and DHA, which are anti-inflammatory. Research shows that taking a high dose of fish oils (3 grams a day) produces a long-term improvement in joint pain and stiffness. Taking fish oil alone, without making any changes to the diet, can bring about improvements. You need to take a daily dose of fish oil for at least three to six months for it to be effective.
GAMMALINOLENIC ACID (GLA)	Found in evening primrose oil, borage seed (starflower) oil and blackcurrant seed oil, GLA is another kind of essential fatty acid. It converts to a prostaglandin called E1, known to have an anti-inflammatory effect. Taking 6 grams a day may help reduce morning stiffness and other symptoms.
ANTIOXIDANTS	Antioxidants are nutrients which scavenge dangerous free radicals in the body and are anti-inflammatory. Antioxidants include Vitamin E and selenium. Rheumatoid arthritis causes inflamed joints, which depletes the joints of vitamin E. A daily intake of 600 iu a day has been shown to help rheumatoid arthritis.
VITAMIN B_5	In rheumatoid arthritis there may be a deficiency of vitamin B_5 (also known as pantothenic acid.) It aids tissue repair. Some nutritionally orientated doctors suggest 1,000 mg of vitamin B_5 to help with morning stiffness, general disability and pain.
VITAMIN B_6	Helps reduce swelling and joint stiffness.
VITAMIN C	Useful if you are taking aspirin, as aspirin depletes the body of vitamin C. Vitamin C can be low in rheumatoid arthritis, possibly because of free radical activity in inflamed areas. Vitamin C is a free radical scavenger and also necessary for cartilage and bone formation. It also promotes the absorption of iron.
IRON	Anaemia may occur in people with rheumatoid arthritis. Follow your doctor's recommendations for taking iron supplements to prevent anaemia.
CALCIUM WITH VITAMIN D	Calcium is important for people with arthritis, especially women who are at risk of developing osteoporosis. Take calcium citrate or chelated calcium. Vitamin D, which you can get from sun exposure and oily fish, helps you body absorb calcium.
ZINC	Zinc metabolism is altered in rheumatoid arthritis and patients are often low in zinc. Working with other nutrients, zinc also has a role to play in reducing inflammation.
SELENIUM	There is a relationship between low levels of the trace element selenium and rheumatoid arthritis. People with the condition seem to have an abnormality in the metabolism of selenium.

DIETARY SUPPLEMENTS FOR OSTEOARTHRITIS

CALCIUM WITH VITAMIN D	Calcium is necessary for building and maintaining strong bones. It is important for people with arthritis, especially women who are at risk of developing osteoporosis. Take calcium citrate or chelated calcium. Vitamin D helps your body absorb calcium. You get it from exposure to sunshine and eating oily fish or cod-liver oil.
GLUCOSAMINE SULPHATE	This is derived from sea shells and contains a building block needed for the repair of joint cartilage. Symptoms may be lessened and damaged joints repaired if you take 500 mg three times a day.
CHONDROITIN SULPHATE	Levels of chondroitin sulphate may be reduced in joint cartilage affected by osteoarthritis and possibly other forms of arthritis. It may help restore joint function. Glucosamine sulphate and chondroitin sulphate can be taken in combination.
VITAMIN B_6	Is needed to help the absorption of glucosamine sulphate and chondroitin sulphate.
ANTIOXIDANTS	Those who eat high levels of antioxidants show a much slower rate of joint deterioration, particularly in the knees. Vitamin E, 400–600 iu a day, has been shown to reduce the symptoms of osteoarthritis. Pycnogenols have a similar effect.
IRON WITH VITAMIN C	Taking painkillers such as aspirin and non-steroidal inflammatory drugs (NSAIDs) can eventually cause stomach ulcers, which can lead to bleeding and anaemia. Increase your iron intake in your meals, as well as vitamin C, which will help your body absorb iron. If necessary your doctor may prescribe iron supplements.
BORON	Boron affects calcium metabolism, and a link between boron deficiency and arthritis has been suggested. When 6 mg of boron is taken daily for two months, it may relieve symptoms of osteoarthritis. However, boron can increase oestrogen levels, so limit boron supplements to 1 mg per day. Sources include bee pollen and kelp.
MAGNESIUM	Needed for the maintenance of healthy bones.
FISH OILS	As with rheumatoid arthritis (see facing page), fish oils may help reduce symptoms of osteoarthritis.
ZINC	Needed for cross-linking and regeneration of connective tissue in cartilage.
NIACINAMIDE	This is a form of vitamin B_3. High doses (250 mg 4–16 times a day) can help increase joint mobility, improve muscle strength and decrease fatigue.
D-PHENYLALALINE	An amino acid used to treat chronic pain, with variable effectiveness.

Exercise

*E*xercise is one of the most important things you can do. It is effective in combating the symptoms and progress of arthritic conditions. It protects against loss of joint function, keeps joints and muscles working, and helps prevent disability.

A good exercise programme strengthens muscles, increases mobility and reduces joint pain and stiffness. It helps control weight and contributes to a greater sense of wellbeing through the release of endorphins. Weight-bearing excercises increase bone density. If you don't exercise, you'll lose muscle strength, and your joints will become more unstable and painful. Inactivity often increases the symptoms of arthritis, and if this leads to weight gain, problems will be worse.

How much and what exercise you do depends on what type of arthritis you have. Even if many of your joints are affected, you still need to exercise. Be cautious, however, about exercising when you are having a flare-up – only do gentle range-of-motion exercises. If possible, have an exercise programme tailor-made to your needs by a physiotherapist. It is best to exercise when you're having the least pain and stiffness and your medication is having the most effect.

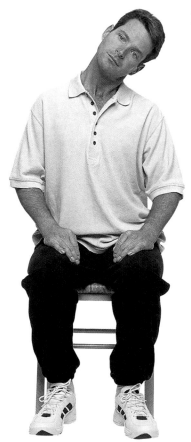

Neck Sideways Bend

To stretch the neck muscles and loosen up tightness.
1. Sitting straight in an upright chair, bend your neck slowly to one side, trying to touch your shoulder with your ear.
2. Straighten your neck, then repeat the other side.
3. Repeat the sequence five to ten times.

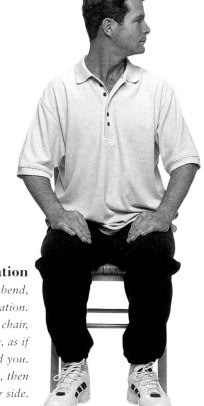

Neck Rotation

Has all the benefits of the sideways bend, and is also good for general circulation.
1. Sit up straight in an upright chair, slowly rotate your neck to one side, as if you were trying to look behind you.
2. Straighten your neck, then repeat on the other side.
3. Repeat the sequence five times.

WHAT TYPES OF EXERCISE ARE BEST FOR ARTHRITIS?

Find out more

Physiotherapy and
   exercise   118–119
Exercise   150–151

There are three types of exercise that are ideal for arthritis sufferers:
- Stretching or range-of-motion (ROM)
- Strengthening
- Aerobic or endurance

They each have a different function, and should not be substituted for each other. You should also pay attention to your body's natural limitations – no advantage will be gained from pushing too hard.

Stretching exercises gently move your joints through their full range of movement as far as they can go. This type of exercise helps maintain joint movement, relieves stiffness and increases flexibility. Stretching exercises should be done twice a day, with periods of rest.

Strengthening exercises are useful when you have lost strength in particular joints. They require repetition to achieve their aim.

Aerobic exercise improves your cardiovascular system and helps to boost your metabolism.

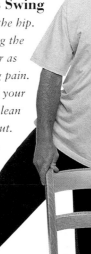

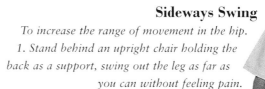

Sideways Swing

To increase the range of movement in the hip.
1. Stand behind an upright chair holding the back as a support, swing out the leg as far as you can without feeling pain.
2. Keep the other leg straight and hold your body upright. Do not allow your body to lean away from the leg you are swinging out.
3. Repeat five to ten times on each side.

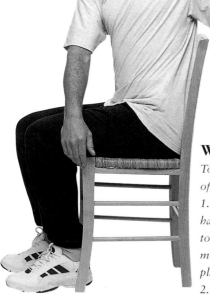

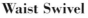

Waist Swivel

To improve the mobility of the waist.
1. Sit up straight in an upright chair with your arms hanging down on either side of the chair. Swivel the top half of your body round to the left hand side, moving your left arm over the back of the chair and placing your left hand over your right thigh.
2. Repeat five to ten times on each side.

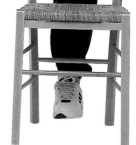

Exercise

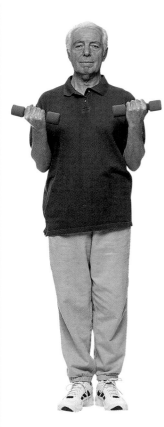

Always begin your strengthening exercises slowly with small weights.

• Strengthening and muscle-conditioning exercises are useful when you have lost strength in particular joints. They contract the muscle around the joint without actually moving the joint itself, thus increasing muscle strength. Start with muscle-strengthening exercises once a day, contracting a muscle for one or two seconds. As you get stronger, gradually build this up so that you are holding for a count of six seconds, then relax and repeat four times, twice a day.

• Aerobic or endurance exercises improve your overall function, promote cardiovascular fitness, increase bone strength and reduce fatigue. They help reduce inflammation in the joints and keep your weight down. Aerobic exercises are more active, such as walking, running, swimming, aerobic dancing, aquatics, or cycling. Aim to do this kind of exercise for 20 minutes two to three times a week.

Getting the most out of exercise

• Don't expect miracles immediately. If you have already lost some function in your joints, it can take a while to regain it.

• Begin to exercise by spending some time on movements that will stretch and loosen tight muscles, tendons and ligaments.

• Start with easy, range-of-motion exercises.

• Add low-impact aerobics when you feel ready.

• If you do exercises that you enjoy, you're more likely to stick with it.

• Rest when you need to. Get the balance right between exercise and rest.

• Expect some normal exercise discomfort. But always stop if you feel any pain.

How much exercise should you do?

It depends on how fit you are and how bad your arthritis is. Ideally, you should do some kind of endurance exercise twice a week and stretching exercises every day. You may feel tired, but a little endurance exercise such as a short walk is likely to make you feel less fatigued.

However, you can exercise too much. If you have more pain two hours after exercising than you did before, do less next time. Warning signs that you are doing too much include unusual or persistent fatigue, swollen joints or decreased range of motion. If your joints become painful, inflamed or red – STOP.

Exercises suitable for arthritis

Walking: This is an ideal exercise for people with arthritis. It is weight-bearing and uses most of the body's major muscles. Walking is easy to incorporate into your daily routine, it puts little strain on the joints and muscles, and it can also help you lose weight.

If you do hill walking, it can help build up the muscles in your legs and thighs, which in turn can stablize the joints in your legs, especially the knees. There is evidence that taking part in a supervised walking programme can alleviate the pain associated with osteoarthritis of the knees.

Spend around 10 to 15 minutes doing warm up exercises – gently stretching the muscles of your arms and legs. Start walking at an easy pace for about five minutes, increasing your speed gradually to a brisk pace. Try and maintain this pace for around 15 to 20 minutes. For the final 5 minutes, slow down again. At the end, stretch for another 5 to 10 minutes to help keep your muscles loose.

If you forget to stretch and begin to feel pain, you could be put off.

If you haven't done much exercise before, start out slowly and gradually build up your distance. Start with a 15 to 30 minute walk, three times a week. As you get fitter, you could walk for longer, adding hills to the route. Don't push yourself if it hurts.

It does not take long to see improvements. If you walk regularly, you should notice a difference in just a month. You may find that you weigh less, have more energy and sleep better.

Even if you do not weigh less, you may look slimmer as your muscles tighten up. You will also have the satisfaction of knowing you are doing something to alleviate arthritic pain. If you make walking a regular habit, you are more likely to stick to it.

Exercising in water: Water takes the weight off your body so that you can do more with less pain.

Swimming is excellent as it exercises your whole body and the water carries your weight. If your local hospital has a warm hydrotherapy pool, ask your doctor to refer you. Many council swimming pools offer aquarobic classes with qualified teachers. If you can find someone else with arthritis to go with, it may be more fun. Be careful not to overdo it in the water.

Golf: If you enjoy golf but have arthritis in your hands you can build up the grips of your clubs with foam pads to reduce the pressure on the joints. Instead of carrying your bag, rent a cart. Make sure that you do plenty of warm-up exercises, which should include stretching your back, hips and shoulders and range-of-motion exercises for your elbows, wrists and hands. Taking a hot bath or shower before playing can also help you feel more flexible.

Other good forms of exercise include cycling, dance therapy, t'ai chi and yoga.

Exercising with other people

Ask your local arthritis organization if there's an exercise programme in your area. Many people find exercising with a group an enjoyable experience as well as a healthy one.

Arthritis doesn't necessarily mean giving up the sports that you enjoy such as golf, but ask your doctor for advice. Always do warm-up exercises before your begin.

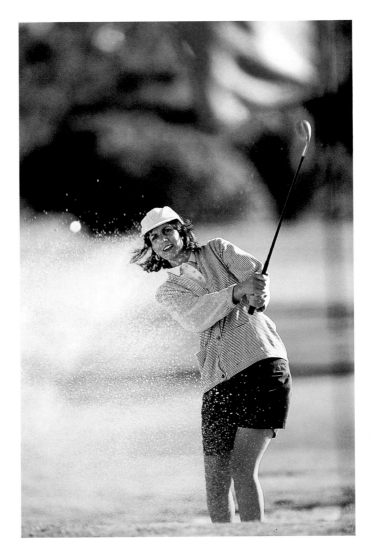

Aids and gadgets

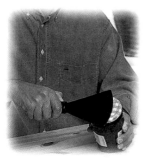

Aids that are placed over a lid enable you to get a good grip and will ease the pain and frustration of opening jars.

A long-handled dustpan and brush will make housework less of a chore.

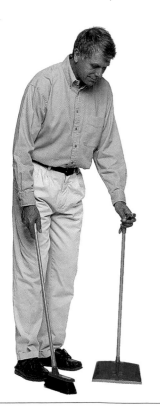

No matter how your arthritis affects you, there is an aid, gadget or piece of equipment that can make your life easier. The range is vast and they are easier to obtain than ever – you can buy many gadgets in high-street stores or through specialist mail-order catalogues. (See Useful Addresses at the end of the book.)

Before paying for larger items, seek the advice of an occupational therapist from the social services department of your local council. They will visit your home, advise you on what aids and equipment you need, and show you how to use them. Some items, such as grab rails for example, may be provided free of charge. You can sometimes borrow equipment from the social services department or your local hospital.

Help from social services

Your general practitioner will need to tell the authorities how your disability affects you. You should arrange for an assessment from both an occupational therapist and a social worker. An occupational therapist will assess you for aids and equipment, and advise what is most suitable in your case. A social worker will assess what care package you need. This may involve visits from a care assistant who can undertake basic housework, food preparation and shopping. You may also be eligible for a service that brings meals to your home.

If your home needs to be adapted, this is done on the recommendation of the occupational therapist. For costly structural alterations, you may be eligible for a grant.

Gadgets for daily activities in the home

• A reaching aid is a long stick with tongs at the top. It helps you reach things without having to bend or stretch so that you can pick things up from the floor or grasp light objects from shelves and cupboards.

• Plugs with handles will help you to get a good grip. If existing sockets are too low for you, ask an electrician to move them higher up the wall, at your waist level, so that they are easier to reach.

• If the light switches are too fiddly, have them replaced by large rocker-action switches. Or have an electrician install a pullcord in every room.

• Have a thermostat fitted to keep the room at a constant temperature. This saves having to adjust knobs and dials.

• Key holders and knob turners can be attached to keys and knobs to give you a good firm grip and longer leverage. Lever type door handles are easier to use than knobs.

• Tap turners have long handles which give extra leverage and can be turned by using the back of the hand, elbow or wrist.

• Attach a basket below the letter box so that you do not have to bend down to pick up the mail.

Kitchen equipment

• Perching stools enable you to sit down when working.

• Kettle tippers help you to avoid lifting hot, heavy teapots and kettles.

• Devices are available to l help you open jars and tins.

- Saucepans and cooking pots should have a handle at both sides. Use a chip basket inside a saucepan to make draining vegetables easier and safer.
- Labour-saving machines such as an electric food processor, an automatic washing machine or a dishwasher can all help to make your life much easier.
- Spike boards hold food steady and leave your hands free and hooped potato peelers are easy on the wrist. Mixing bowls can be kept steady on anti-slip mats, or buy one with suction pads.
- Use a trolley rather than a heavy tray.
- Look for two-handed mugs and easy-grip cutlery.

Bathrooms and toilets
- A raised toilet seat is useful for stiff knees and hips. Grab rails placed at the side of the toilet make it easier to get on and off. There are also free-standing toilet frames.
- Commodes can be placed by the bed so that you do not have to go to the bathroom. Portable urinals can be used while lying in bed or sitting on the edge.
- A small step, grab rails and non-slip mats all make getting in and out of the bath easier.
- Mechanical bath lifts and hoists make it possible to have a bath independently.
- Taking a shower can be easier if you have a shower seat. Some firms specialize in showers designed for disabled people.

Equipment for getting around the house
- Walking aids include walking sticks, elbow crutches and walking frames.
- Stairlifts enable you to glide up and down stairs.
- Grab rails on both sides of steps make them easier. If you cannot manage steps, you may need a ramp.

- A wheelchair needs plenty of space to move between rooms and turn around so you may need to make alterations to your home, such as wider doorways or ramps.

Furniture
- Chairs should have a firm back and armrests. You can raise the height of low chairs by putting blocks under the legs. "Riser" chairs have an electrically operated mechanism to help you on to your feet.
- Beds should be the right height as a low bed can be hard to get out of. The mattress should be firm enough to support your spine without sagging. Adjustable beds enable you to choose the most comfortable position just by the touch of a button. Twin beds have dual controls, so that each partner has the freedom to be in the position they want. This system can help relieve arthritic pain and give you a good night's sleep. A "leglifter" helps lift weak or painful legs into bed.

Plugs with handles will help you to get a good grip. If sockets are hard to reach, think about having them moved up.

Look out for devices that will help you to open medicine jars and bottles.

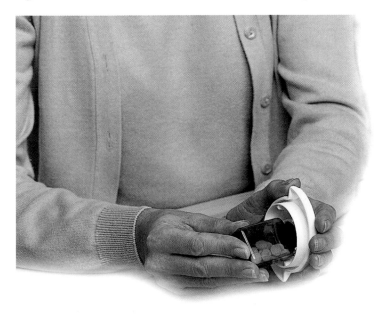

Glossary

Acupoints – specific points along the meridians at which the flow of qi or chi, the fundamental life-energy of the universe, can be stimulated.

Analgesic – a pain-relieving substance or drug.

Ankylosing spondylitis – a form of arthritis in which the joints of the spine gradually stiffen and lock rigid.

Anti-inflammatory – drugs designed to reduce inflammation and ease pain.

Arthroscope – a fibre-optic instrument passed through a small cut in the flesh to enable a surgeon to examine a joint.

Cartilage – the tough and slippery covering at the end of bones where they meet to form joints.

Chi – another spelling of qi, the universal life-energy in Traditional Chinese Medicine.

Corticosteroids – hormones produced by the body and also synthesized for use as anti-inflammatories.

Heberden's nodes – bony growths on the fingers, a sign of osteoarthritis.

Juvenile rheumatoid arthritis – one of the several types of arthritis that occur in children.

Ligament – a band of tough, fibrous tissue that supports bones at a joint and controls the way in which they can move.

Lupus – an autoimmune disease; also known as systemic lupus erythematosus.

Meridian – a channel that runs through the body carrying the life-force, qi or chi. There are 14 main meridians.

Osteoarthritis – the most common form of degenerative arthritis, in which healthy cartilage starts to crack and flake.

Osteophytes – bony, spur-like growths on or around the vertebrae. Osteophytes are a feature of osteoarthritis.

Prana – the fundamental life-energy of the universe in Ayurvedic medicine, the traditional Indian system of healing. Also known as qi or chi in Traditional Chinese Medicine.

Qi – in Traditional Chinese Medicine, the fundamental life-energy of the universe, also known as chi; the equivalent of prana in Ayurvedic medicine.

Rheumatoid arthritis – the most common form of inflammatory arthritis, in which the synovial membrane thickens.

Synovial fluid – a clear fluid produced by the synovial membrane that lubricates the joints.

Tendon – a tough band of tissue connecting muscle to bone.

Tendonitis – Inflammation of a tendon.

Tincture – a herbal remedy prepared by chopping or grinding up a plant and soaking it in an alcohol solution. The mixture is left to stand for several weeks, then the liquid is strained off and taken by mouth.

Tisane – an infusion of a herbal remedy prepared in a way similar to brewing tea. The herbs are infused in hot water in a teapot for about 10 minutes, the liquid is poured off and drunk hot or cold.